# MENTAL ILLNESS IN THE FAMILY
## ISSUES AND TRENDS

*Mental Illness in the Family* traces the development of treatment approaches with families of the mentally ill over the past three decades. The essays in this book reflect, from a number of perspectives, the work of clinicians currently dealing with families in a variety of settings. Topics covered include patients' views on programs for the mentally ill, the needs of families coming to terms with the mental illness of a family member, 'the forgotten sibling,' the concept of grief, the confusion that a family member can experience when dealing simultaneously with the mental health and criminal justice systems, and the effect of parental mental illness on young children.

This volume will be of particular interest to social workers, clinical psychiatrists, psychologists, and other mental health professionals who work with individuals and families who have been affected by major mental illness.

BEVERLEY ABOSH is Vice President of Professional Services and Social Worker-in-Chief at the Clarke Institute of Psychiatry.
APRIL COLLINS is a social worker with the Clinical Investigation Unit and First Episode Psychosis Program at the Clarke Institute of Psychiatry.

EDITED BY BEVERLEY ABOSH AND
APRIL COLLINS

# Mental Illness in the Family: Issues and Trends

UNIVERSITY OF TORONTO PRESS
Toronto Buffalo London

© University of Toronto Press Incorporated 1996
Toronto Buffalo London
Printed in Canada

ISBN 0-8020-2905-1 (cloth)
ISBN 0-8020-7412-x (paper)

Printed on acid-free paper

**Canadian Cataloguing in Publication Data**

Main entry under title:

Mental illness in the family

Expanded and updated papers originally presented at
a conference entitled Mental illness in the family
hosted by the Dept. of Social Work, Clarke Institute
of Psychiatry, Toronto, Nov. 7, 1991.

ISBN 0-8020-2905-1 (bound)
ISBN 0-8020-7412-x (pbk.)

1. Mentally ill. – Family relationships – Congresses.
2. Mental illness – Congresses.   3. Family
psychotherapy – Congresses.   I. Abosh, Beverley.
II. Collins, April.   III. Clarke Institute of
Psychiatry, Social Work Dept.

RC455.4.F3M45 1996       616.89      C95-932844-0

University of Toronto Press acknowledges the financial assistance to its pub-
lishing program of the Canada Council and Ontario Arts Council.

# Contents

# Acknowledgments

This book is the culmination of a shared vision about patients and their families, their hopes and their struggle with mental illness. We are grateful to everyone who contributed to the book.

We would like to thank Dr Paul Garfinkel for his generous support of the project. Our thanks go to Elizabeth Lamb, who gave unstintingly of her time and patience in the preparation of the manuscript. Finally, we are also indebted to Diane Thomas and the staff of the Clarke library.

# Contributors

**Beverley Abosh, MSW, CSW**
Vice-President Professional Services and Social Worker-in-Chief, Clarke Insitute of Psychiatry; Social Work Practice Professor, Faculty of Social Work; and Assistant Professor, Department of Psychiatry, Faculty of Medicine, University of Toronto

**Leona L. Bachrach, Ph.D.**
Research Professor of Psychiatry, Maryland Psychiatric Research Center, University of Maryland Department of Psychiatry; Visiting Professor, Department of Psychiatry, Faculty of Medicine, University of Toronto

**Tatyana Barankin, MD, FRCP(C), Dipl. Child Psychiatry**
Assistant Professor, Department of Psychiatry, Faculty of Medicine, University of Toronto; Head, Clinic for Children at Risk, Child and Family Studies Centre, Clarke Institute of Psychiatry

**Christina Bartha, MSW, CSW**
Chief Social Worker, Mood/Anxiety Division, Clarke Institute of Psychiatry

**Dale Butterill, MSW**
Coordinator, Community Linkage Program, Clarke Institute of Psychiatry

**April Collins, MSW, CSW**
Social Worker, Clinical Investigation Unit and First Episode Psychosis Program, Clarke Institute of Psychiatry

**Dave Denberg, MSW, CSW**
Social Worker, General Psychiatry Division, Clarke Institute of Psychiatry

**Luis F. Goncalves, MSW, CSW**
Senior Family Counsellor and Intake Coordinator, Family Services Association – Municipality of Peel

**Myrna Greenberg, MSW**
Social Worker, Child and Family Studies Centre, Clarke Institute of Psychiatry

**Agnes B. Hatfield, PhD**
Professor Emeritus, Unviersity of Maryland, College Park, Maryland

**Debra MacRae, MSW, CSW**
Social Worker, Family Court Clinic, Clarke Institute of Psychiatry

**Jane Paterson, MSW, CSW**
Chief Social Worker, Continuing Care Division, Clarke Institute of Psychiatry

**Marlene Swirsky, MSW, CSW**
Chief Social Worker, Metropolitan Toronto Forensic Service (METFORS), Clarke Institute of Psychiatry

**John Trainor, MSW**
Director, Community Support and Research Unit, Queen Street Mental Health Centre; Lecturer, Department of Psychiatry, Faculty of Medicine, University of Toronto

**Elizabeth Tuters, MSW, CSW**
Social Worker, Hincks Centre for Children's Mental Health; Director, Toronto Child Psychotherapy Program

**Froma Walsh, PhD**
Professor, School of Social Service Administration and Department of Psychiatry; Co-Director, Center for Family Health, University of Chicago

MENTAL ILLNESS IN THE FAMILY:
ISSUES AND TRENDS

# Introduction

The idea for this book originated at a 1991 conference entitled 'Mental Illness in the Family,' hosted by the Department of Social Work at the Clarke Institute of Psychiatry. Since the conference was held to commemorate the Clarke's twenty-fifth anniversary, it seemed appropriate to reflect on clinical practice and to examine how approaches to families affected by mental illness have evolved over the past twenty-five years.

There have been significant changes in the delivery of mental health services and in the treatment of mental illness in the past three decades. The deinstitutionalization movement of the late 1950s and early 1960s, which resulted in many patients being discharged from large institutions and brought into the community, dramatically shifted the locus of care. Increasingly families were being called upon to provide care for their mentally ill relatives. Neuroleptic drugs were becoming available at about the same time as developments in psychoanalytic thinking and family therapy were emerging. Optimism about treatment possibilities abounded. Many mental health professionals embraced the exciting field of family therapy, which was so full of promise, seemingly for all forms of mental illness. Family therapy was fascinating, frustrating, and intellectually stimulating, but ultimately disappointing. When families were faced with a severe and debilitating illness such as schizophrenia, even the most insightful, perceptive interpretations were not helpful. Mental health professionals, unwittingly perhaps, caused much grief to families by adopting what many perceived to be an attitude of blame. Families were too often viewed as causative agents in the etiology of the illness and as 'noxious' influences on patients. They were frequently regarded as 'unidentified patients' who were themselves in need of therapeutic change.

More recent research in the neurosciences indicating that schizophrenia and affective disorders have strong biochemical and genetic roots has been greeted with relief, and indeed with optimism, by families of the mentally ill. The evidence of biological roots of mental illness has challenged many of the original assumptions regarding families as etiological agents. Families have discovered their collective voice and have lobbied hard to gain respect within the mental health system.

The relationship between mental health professionals and families continues to undergo significant change. Families want to be seen as allies, not adversaries, and need acknowledgment of their strengths. They also need specific information about their relatives' illness, access to resources, and assurances of continuity of care. As well, all families, however strong, have certain needs for support in times of stress and crisis. They require the understanding that caring for a mentally ill relative can be difficult, exhausting, and stressful. They need professionals to be aware of the demands of caregiving.

This book includes a number of papers originally presented at the 1991 conference. They have been expanded and updated to reflect the work of clinicians who are currently dealing with families in a variety of settings and from a number of different perspectives. We are fortunate to present here essays by our three distinguished keynote speakers. In chapter 1, 'What Do Patients Say about Program Planning? Perspectives from the Patient-Authored Literature,' Dr Leona Bachrach presents patients' views on program planning for the mentally ill. This essay is particularly timely in an era of increasing consumer advocacy and involvement in mental health planning. In chapter 2, 'Families and Mental Illness: What Have We Learned?' Dr Froma Walsh outlines the developments in family therapy over the past three decades. She emphasizes the importance of adopting a biopsychosocial orientation in treatment and the need to shift from viewing families as pathogenic influences to involving them as valued resources. In chapter 5, 'Out of the Ashes of Mental Illness ... A New Life,' Dr Agnes B. Hatfield urges mental health professionals to be cognizant of the family's need to come to terms with having a relative with a devastating mental illness. She stresses the importance of adopting a holistic, long-term view that takes into account the survival of the family as a unit, as well as providing a support system for the ill relative.

The remaining essays reflect the variety of ways in which mental health professionals work with families. Chapters 4 and 5 deal with the changing relationships among consumers, families, and the mental health system. John Trainor looks at the growing political power of family organizations. Dale Butterill and Jane Paterson propose a three-stage model that allows for different types of family interventions, depending on the needs of the family. The authors contend that the needs of families living with chronic mental illness change over time. They argue for a clearly articulated theory of family functioning that would encompass a synthesis of three important perspectives – those of the family, the consumer, and the mental health professional.

In chapter 6, Marlene Swirsky discusses the confusing, and often frightening, experiences a family can encounter when dealing with both the mental health system and the criminal justice system.

Chapter 7 discusses grief, a significant and frequently unrecognized experience for families dealing with the serious mental illness of a relative. April Collins argues cogently that, despite the increased attention given to families of the seriously mentally ill, the needs addressed are commonly those associated with stabilization of an acute psychotic episode. Families are not often given the opportunity to mourn the loss of hopes and dreams they may have had for a child afflicted with a chronic illness.

Chapter 8 explores sibling relationships, an area that is frequently neglected in clinical practice and in the literature. Dave Denberg examines both the historical and the current literature on siblings of the mentally ill. He concludes that sibling relationships are more complex and significant than was previously thought, that psychiatric illness intrudes on sibling bonds, and that they can have a lifelong influence, often independent of parental relationships.

The impact of parental affective disorders on families, is addressed by Tatyana Barankin and Myrna Greenberg in chapter 9. Interest among professionals in evaluating the consequences of parental affective disorders on children is a fairly recent phenomenon. This essay reviews the literature regarding the 'risk' and 'protective' factors for children when a parent suffers a recurrent affective disorder. The authors argue that efforts should be directed towards increasing resilience in all family members, and suggest a variety of cognitive and psychoeducational approaches.

Chapters 10, 11, and 12 deal more specifically with how mental illness in a parent can affect younger children. Christina Bartha and Luis Goncalves address the dilemma confronting professionals when mental illness interferes with a person's parenting ability and when termination of parental rights is a consideration. Their essay provides a review of the literature that considers the impact of mental illness on parenting capacity and presents a structured model of assessment and clinical decision making.

Debra MacRae and Elizabeth Tuters provide clinical examples of how a sensitive and supportive psychotherapeutic approach can be effective in dealing with difficult family situations. MacRae's essay on therapy with a youngster who can no longer live with his parents reminds us of what can be accomplished in the context of a caring therapeutic relationship. Tuters's essay on the mother–infant relationship draws attention to the need for a supportive network for high-risk families as well as for intensive mother–infant therapy.

This book addresses some of the current issues in working with families when a member is suffering from mental illness. Advances in biological research, and the growing acceptance by mental health professionals of the family's need for information, have altered and enhanced our clinical practice. Increasingly, families are becoming involved with mental health professionals in new partnerships. The mental health system in general has become more responsive to the needs of individual patients and families. Recent shifts in mental health policy (Ontario Ministry of Health, 1993) have reflected the importance of families and the emerging power of family organizations.

The realignment of relationships among families, consumers, and mental health professionals has been productive. Many educational programs have been developed, and the importance of ready access to community resources has been stressed. However, as beneficial as these developments have been, there is concern that the pendulum has perhaps swung too far. In spite of recent progress it is necessary to guard against a form of clinical reductionism that would deny families and patients the opportunity to explore their inner worlds in therapy. Psychoeducation and psychotherapy are not mutually exclusive. Working with families on both the instrumental and the psychological level is necessary for of comprehensive and compassionate care.

BEVERLEY ABOSH AND APRIL COLLINS

REFERENCE

Ontario Ministry of Health. (1993). *Putting people first: The reform of mental health services in Ontario.* Toronto: Author.

# What Do Patients Say about Program Planning? Perspectives from the Patient-Authored Literature[*]

## LEONA L. BACHRACH

Persons who are or have been patients in the mental health system have for some years been writing about their experiences as service recipients. They are perforce experts in the field of mental health program planning, and their contributions are often frank, articulate, and exceedingly sensitive. These writings contain important clues and information from which mental health program planners might take direction. Yet surprisingly little note has been taken of the patient-authored literature in the development of program initiatives for mentally ill individuals.

This essay examines the patient-authored literature and seeks to establish points of agreement between patient-authors and professionals who design and plan mental health programs. Are the pet planning concepts that professionals embrace reinforced or contradicted in patients' writings? And has anything that is important to patient-authors been overlooked by professionals?

To answer these questions, I employ three basic concepts that have become increasingly popular in professional program-planning circles in recent years: that treatment resistance among patients ('difficult patienthood') has more than one source; that disabilities accompanying severe mental illness are complex and multivariate; and that service planning for mentally ill persons should, ideally, be tailored to the needs of each individual member of the patient population.

These three concepts are, perhaps, more accurately described as 'conceptual fields,' for each is intricately intertwined with other principles and

---

[*] An earlier version of this chapter appeared in Jeffrey R. Bedell (Ed.), *Psychological Assessment and Treatment of Persons with Severe Mental Disorder* (pp. 75–91). Washington, DC: Taylor & Francis 1994.

concepts. Together they generate the framework for this analysis, which reviews patient-authored writings retrieved through a Medline search of periodical literature published over the past decade. Earlier writings by patients that seem especially relevant have also been examined, as have patient-authored writings from miscellaneous sources – the so-called fugitive literature consisting of letters, newspaper clippings, agency publications, conference proceedings, and other unindexed statements.

This essay does not purport to be a comprehensive review of patient-authored literature. The focus here is specifically on program-planning issues as they are discussed in that literature. Nor is this essay concerned with the politics of the patient-rights movement or with advocacy for mental patients, important as those matters are. Instead, this essay aims to take a small step towards bridging the gap between the perspectives of patient-authors and those of professional program designers. In other words, it is an attempt to assess what outsiders looking in may learn from insiders speaking out about issues in mental health program planning and service delivery.

Given that patients' own words carry the greatest impact, patient-authored writings are directly quoted throughout this review. These writings are often poetic and lyrical, as the late Jack Weinberg (1978, p. 25) noted when he wrote about 'the words of the emotionally ill ... the poetry of the anguished mentality.'

By way of example, a patient at the Rhode Island Institute of Mental Health (1984) who signs his name as Tom writes:

Getting out of here
And into something
Like work
Or something payable
Like caddying
I've had some good days
And some rainy ones
Sometimes it would
Break your heart
To see the rain
When it comes
But to be able
To hang around and hope
Helps a lot
But to sit

And be incarcerated
Almost drives you
To be tapioca

Another patient at the same hospital (ibid.), who signs his name as Robert, writes:

Fill my mind with knowledge
Fill my body with definition
Fill my life with total well being
Fill my pockets with money
Fill my nerves with relaxation
Fill myself with the old me

## Planning Concepts

Mental health program planning today – at least on paper if not in actual fact – is generally influenced by three interrelated factors: first, emerging ideas about what makes a patient resistant to treatment, non-compliant, or 'difficult'; second, our understanding of the concept of disability as it affects mentally ill individuals; and, third, our promotion of individualized treatment planning for the members of the patient population.

### Difficult Patienthood

The term 'difficult patient,' which is frequently used to indicate a patient's resistance to treatment or lack of cooperation (Bachrach, Talbott, & Meyerson, 1987), is inherently stigmatizing. It is also in some ways meaningless, since 'all patients who have been designated as having a psychiatric condition are expected to be problems to themselves as well as to their respective environments, which includes the psychiatrist who comes into contact with them' (Chrzanowski, 1980, p. 27). For these reasons, recent literature has discussed both patient and extra-patient sources of difficult patienthood.

Three interrelated kinds of precipitants are typically discussed (Bachrach, Talbott, & Meyerson, 1987). First, difficult patienthood may be attributed to the patient him- or herself: to certain behaviours, characteristics, or attributes that distinguish that patient from other 'non-difficult' patients. Neill (1979) reports that, as compared with their non-difficult counterparts, difficult patients tend to be more demanding, more puzzling, less likely to evoke empathy, more dangerous to themselves and others, more attention-seeking and manipulative, more likely to polarize staff, more technically difficult as psychiatric cases, and more likely to misuse medication.

Second, difficult patienthood may be attributed to the clinician who works with the patient, to the clinician's biases or expectations, or to the 'rules' that clinicians often impose. Examples might include stipulations that the illness be treatable and preferably curable; that the patient be fully cooperative; and that the patient regard his or her condition as something that must be changed (Jeffery, 1979). When a patient does not meet these expectations, the clinican may well view that individual as a difficult patient.

It is, however, exceedingly difficult in practice to separate the first and second sources of difficult patienthood. There is increasing consensus in the literature that the distinguishing personal characteristics, attributes, and behaviours of so-called difficult patients are only contextually troublesome: that they may be necessary, but they are not sufficient, for the definition of difficult patienthood (Bachrach, Talbott, & Meyerson, 1987). A particular patient's behaviours or attributes are thus difficult only when they are perceived as such by clinicians, administrators, or service planners.

Third, difficult patienthood may be attributed to the service system itself, or more precisely to deficiencies within that system. When the service system lacks sufficient motivation or resources to provide continuity of care and comprehensive care, it tends to build a protective shield around itself. Harris and Bergman (1986–7, p. 203) have introduced the concept of the 'narcissistically vulnerable system' to describe the defensive postures assumed by service structures that 'are primarily concerned with maintaining an often fragile sense of self-esteem.' It is not uncommon for the service system to identify as difficult patients those whom it will not or cannot serve, or whom it will not or cannot treat, and thereby absolve itself of the obligation to care for these individuals.

These three sources of difficult patienthood are highly interdependent (Bachrach, Talbott, & Meyerson, 1987). The most critical point concerning them is that it takes more than just the patient to make a 'difficult patient.' It takes a context as well – a context that consists of both clinician variables and system variables.

Patients' Views
The three sources of difficult patienthood are fully acknowledged in the

patient-authored literature, often with great insight. As for the first, patient-authored writings frankly admit that patients at times exhibit behaviours or characteristics that are sufficiently removed from the mainstream that they are troublesome to clinicians, service systems, relatives, and society at large. Indeed, far from denying this, the patient-authored literature frequently implies – and sometimes explicitly states – that such behaviours and characteristics should be considered predictable manifestations of severe and debilitating illness.

Moreover, patient-authors appear to have an unusual talent for demonstrating the interdependence of the first and second sources of difficult patienthood. They frequently observe that patients' troublesome behaviours, attributes, and characteristics must be understood as the flip side of clinicians' attitudes and expectations. Thus, one former patient, Sharp (1988), implores clinicians to recognize and acknowledge their own role in promoting difficult patienthood: 'If you don't like someone, get them a doctor who does like them. Don't just get stonefaced and argumentative, but have the strength to let go. Be more responsive.' Indeed, Sharp, who in her writings frequently addresses clinicians directly in the second person, often employs a bit of irony and humour: 'Doctors, pills are pills, however you slice them, and you have all the control, but only the patient knows if he wants to take one a second time, whether it helps or hurts. You're not veterinarians, so your patients can speak and you will get your best clues by listening to them, and by believing them you will get the truth.'

Similarly, patient-authors often offer direct and convincing illustrations of the relationship between difficult patienthood and system inadequacy. They frequently report personal histories filled with searches for appropriate and responsive programs – programs that are, most often, simply not to be found. Or, if the programs can be found, the barriers to using them are perceived by patients as multiple, subtle, and generally insuperable.

The message here is clear. Patient-authors tell us in no uncertain terms that, if patients are to become more compliant and less burdensome to the system of care, the system must do its part to welcome them and respond to their needs. Indeed, concern with system deficiencies has led one well-known patient-author, Allen (1974), to formulate a patients' bill of rights. Allen, who in the late 1970s served on President Carter's Commission on Mental Health, delivers a strong and persuasive message that is often found in the patient-authored literature: that comprehensive services, full access to care, and individualized treatment, delivered with regard for patients' personhood and dignity, must be made available to mentally ill individuals.

In this connection, Brundage (1983, p. 585) writes: 'The effectiveness in reaching and working with patients rests largely upon the ability of the caregiver to perceive and comprehend how particular patients are experiencing their illnesses ... Meticulous honesty and fairness on the part of the caregiver is important. Sometimes patients ... get even more confused in the face of ambiguity and deception ... Tact and understanding of the patients' distress will go a long way toward increasing self-esteem and feelings of self-worth.'

*Sources of Disability*

A second strong influence on contemporary program planning for mentally ill individuals is the notion of disability. There is a growing awareness today that disability typically derives from more than one source. Although some portion is directly attributable to the illness, other contributing sources include the way in which the individual patient responds to his or her illness and the way in which the system of care and society respond to the patient. These ideas are central in the writings of several British investigators, including Wing and Morris (1981) and Shepherd (1984), who discuss three essential varieties of disability.

Primary Disability
The primary disabilities are those associated with illness per se and consist of psychiatric impairments or dysfunctions that may otherwise be described as symptoms of illness. For example, individuals diagnosed with chronic schizophrenia might exhibit such primary disabilities as lethargy, odd and unacceptable behaviour, a lack of awareness of their handicaps, and disturbances in social relationships. It is typically the appearance of these symptoms of illness or primary disabilities that leads to diagnosis, and, for many individuals, although not for all, to treatment in the mental health care system.

Many patient-authors discuss their primary disabilities openly. Leete (1987), a former patient who is currently program director for education, advocacy, and support at Consumer-Centered Services of Colorado in Denver, describes in vivid language her hallucinations, suspiciousness, and disorganization: 'Sometimes I pace endlessly to relieve the anxiety. I may become frozen in a certain position just because it feels right ... [I] curl up, rock back and forth, pace, or become rigid, at times knowing how bizarre this appears.' And McKay (1986, p. C1), a woman diagnosed as schizophrenic who lives in a shelter for homeless women in Washington, DC, writes: 'I have been a homeless woman for five years. Sometimes I am sharply aware of my surroundings; sometimes I am like a plastic doll, my staring eyes open but unseeing, or I am like a zombie, moving but unfeeling.' A former English teacher, McKay has authored two moving and instructive articles on schizophrenia for the *Washington Post.*

In fact, the importance of accepting one's primary disabilities – one's acknowledgment of illness per se – emerges as a common theme in much of the patient-authored literature. Leete (1987) articulates this idea precisely: 'It was not until I had come to accept my illness that I could seriously devise ways of overcoming it.'

In this connection some, though certainly not all, patient-authors – perhaps because they are willing and able to acknowledge their primary disabilities – do not summarily dismiss the need for pharmacotherapies. The literature frequently acknowledges that medications, appropriately prescribed and monitored, are essential to progress. Leete (1987) writes: 'Despite the embarrassment of troublesome side effects, I now use medication as an adjunct to my other coping mechanisms. However, for many years before I came to realize the role medication could play in the management of my illness, I was caught in a vicious circle. When I was off the medication I couldn't remember how much better I had felt on it, and when I was taking the medication I felt so good that I was convinced I did not need it. Fortunately, through many years of trial and error, I have now learned what medication works best for me and when to take it to minimize side effects.' Similarly, Harris (1988, p. 60), notes: 'I now must take daily medication. I didn't realize until the last time I went off of it how important the medicine is. Without it, I can't function. It's the difference between being insane and sane.'

## Secondary Disability
Wing and Morris (1981) and Shepherd (1984) have written about secondary disabilities that build upon the primary ones. These disabilities result, not from the illness itself, but rather from the experience of illness. Wing has referred to secondary disabilities as 'adverse personal reactions,' and Shepherd (p. 5) aptly notes that 'a major psychiatric episode is a frightening and disturbing experience and its effects may persist long after the primary symptoms have disappeared.' Secondary disabilities, then, represent the individual patient's idiosyncratic response to his or her own illness.

Many patient-authors concur. The notion of secondary disability is clearly expressed in an anonymous article appearing in the *American Journal of Psychiatry*: 'Even if medication can free the schizophrenic patient from some of his torment, the scars of emotional confusion remain, felt perhaps more deeply by a greater sensitivity and vulnerability' (Recovering Patient, 1986, p. 68). Robinson (1983, p. D2), another former patient, offers this description of her secondary disabilities: 'I was pretty terrified at how far I [had] deteriorated into psychosis ... The world of a psychotic is definitely not a pretty one. I remember well the feverish, sleepless nights I spent getting carried away to some magical realm by my own thoughts. My thinking process seemed to me a miracle that could conquer anyone else's. Yet those same thinking processes could overwhelm me into crying oceans of tears over some nostalgic trivia; worse, I could be seized by episodic spasms of sheer unknowable terrors.'

The patient-authored literature in fact contains recurrent references to personal reactions of anger, as exemplified in an article by McGrath (1984, p. 639): 'I sound angry – I guess I am – at the illness for invading my life and making me feel so unsure of myself ... at the medical researchers who now only want to pick and probe into brains or wherever so they can program measurements into their computers while ignoring me, the person ... at all the literature which shrouds schizophrenia in negativity, making any experience connected with it crazy and unacceptable ... at the pharmaceutical industry for being satisfied that their pills keep me "functional" when all the while I feel drugged and unreal to myself. And I'm angry at me for believing and trusting too much in all this information and becoming nothing more than a patient, a victim of some intangible illness. It's no wonder to me anymore why I feel I've lost my self, why my existence seems a waning reflection.' This same article also refers to experiences of fear: 'My illness is a journey of fear, often paralyzing, mostly painful. If only someone could put a band-aid on the wound ... but where? Sometimes I feel I can't stand it any longer.'

Feelings of extreme isolation are commonly expressed. A patient writing in the *New York Times* (Anonymous, 1986, p. C3) asks, 'Can I ever forget that I am schizophrenic? I am isolated and I am alone. I am never real. I play-act my life, touching and feeling only shadows.' And Beeman (1988, p. 4) writes: 'So you end up alone. I think the depression is caused by your isolation, and by the emotional biochemical changes that mental illness causes. It's something you have to experience ... It's a painful, yearning kind of thing. It's torture. You yearn to be part of society, but you're locked into your own private prison and you can't get out. It's a terrible thing.'

Both Wing and Morris (1981) and Shepherd (1984) have noted that the secondary disabilities may present as much of a problem for successful engagement and treatment as do the primary symptoms of the illness itself. From the patients' perspective the critical point regarding these secondary disabilities is that they generally persist, even after the primary symptoms have disappeared.

Tertiary Disability

Wing and Morris (1981) and Shepherd (1984) have discussed tertiary disabilities, or 'social disablements' that are external to the patient. These disabilities come neither from the illness itself nor from personal responses to illness, but rather from societal reactions to mental illness. Leete (1987) provides a particularly succinct and moving description of tertiary disabilities: 'Sadly, in addition to handicaps imposed by our illnesses, the mentally disabled must constantly deal with barriers erected by society as well. Of these, there is none more devastating, discrediting and disabling to an individual recovering from mental illness than stigma. We are denied jobs, unwanted in our communities. We are seen as unattractive, lazy, stupid, unpredictable, and dangerous.'

Some sources of tertiary disability are obvious (for example, inadequate housing, stigma, poverty, unemployment, and marginalization with in society). Yet, serious as these are, we are at least able to name them and, potentially, to consider means for eradicating them. It is the more subtle sources of tertiary disability – the ones for which we have no names – that most worry many professionals involved in mental health program planning. For example, bureaucratic decisions to separate mental health, drug-abuse, and alcoholism services in federal and state agencies may promote unrecognized tertiary disabilities (Bachrach, 1987). Because patients often have multiple problems, they may require services offered in all three classes of agencies. This service fragmentation often discourages comprehensiveness and continuity of care. It may at times even provide a gatekeeping function for agencies by legitimizing their exclusion of certain kinds of patients. This increases patients' vulnerability, and they 'fall through the cracks' in the absence of a central authority to determine where they 'really' belong.

Patient-authors are generally direct in voicing their concern over tertiary disabilities, both the obvious and the more subtle ones. In fact, the literature contains so many excellent examples that one could probably devote an entire review to this subject alone. Rogers (1986), the chairperson of the U.S. National Mental Health Consumers' Association, captures the general sense of that literature in testimony presented before a Senate subcommittee: 'Over the years, I have found that there is very little understanding in the community of the problem of mental illness, and a lot of fear. There's a great deal of stigma, a negative attitude on the part of the public and, unfortunately, in many communities on the part of public officials. There's a feeling that we must sweep this illness under the rug; we must lock the people away; we must not deal with it.'

## Relationships among Disabilities

In many of the examples cited here, it is difficult to differentiate precisely among primary, secondary, and tertiary disabilities. Indeed, the patient-authored literature makes a major contribution in reinforcing the point that these disabilities are separable only in theory and that they are inextricably interwoven in patients' daily lives. The result of this complex interweaving is a milieu filled with pain and despair. The previously cited anonymous author in the *American Journal of Psychiatry* writes: 'During times when I am able to recognize ... [a] need for closeness, yet remain afraid of it, pushing people away while perceiving them as rejecting me, I struggle with incredible pain. It seems that a great chasm spans between myself and that which I want so much and which I try so hard to get. Even as I write these words I am overcome by what seems the impossibility of closing the gap; I must struggle every day not to lose sight of the fact that I am learning and although I feel stagnant at times and overrun by fears both from within and without, it is indeed possible that one day I will achieve that which I seek' (Recovering Patient, 1986, p. 70). The same writer is moved to question the unqualified value of treatment: 'With the struggles back and forth it almost seems questionable at times whether all this is really worth it. There are days when I wonder if it might not be more humane to leave the schizophrenic patient to his own world of unreality, not to make him go through the pain it takes to become a part of humanity.'

### Disability and Difficult Patienthood

Not only do patient-authors document the inextricable link among various sources of disability; they go beyond this to establish that there is also an inescapable relationship between the concepts of disability and difficult patienthood. Patient-authors urge professionals to ask a basic, but perhaps uncomfortable, question: Are patients burdensome to clinicians and to service systems – that is, are they difficult patients – because of their illnesses, their primary disabilities? Or might other circumstances account for patients' lack of cooperation or compliance?

The answer is, of course, a complex one. Certainly, some portion of difficult patienthood resides in illness-related primary symptoms. Yet it seems likely that other major causes of patients' apparent intractability are related to the fact that professionals often expect mentally ill people to behave in ways that complicate their clinical courses and exacerbate their disabilities. Clinicians' expectations, in tandem with service-system deficiencies, often increase patients' secondary and tertiary disabilities and cause them immeasurable pain, a point once again underscored by Leete (1987): 'I have come to believe that mental health clients are not treatment-resistant, as is so often stated, but instead only system-resistant.' Thus, it is not enough to offer patients pharmacotherapies that might reduce their symptoms, that address only their primary disabilities. Those disabilities must be treated, but they are only part of the picture. Similarly, it is not enough to provide patients with therapies and rehabilitative interventions that might reverse their secondary disabilities, that might help them respond more appropriately to their illnesses. These kinds of interventions are certainly important, too; but, once again, they are only part of a larger picture.

The patient-authored literature leaves little doubt, that mental health service systems, in responding to the needs of mentally ill individuals, must also be sensitive to the societal dimensions of illness. The literature strongly supports the notion that service systems must try, as best they can, to mitigate conditions such as service fragmentation, urban gentrification, limited housing, stigma, and lack of health and welfare resources, and even more subtle circumstances that we have not yet named, which profoundly affect the lives of those who are mentally ill.

### Individualized Treatment Planning

A third conceptual area influencing mental health program planning today is our growing understanding of the need for individualized treatments. The fact that those patients who need the most comprehensive and sophisticated care are often given the least individualized treatment has become a source of great concern to many planners, and it is probably accurate to predict that the future success of mental health programs will depend upon our ability to implement the concepts associated with individualized treatment (Bachrach, 1989).

Once again, statements in the patient-authored literature support this notion, often with great poignancy. McKay (1987, p. C1), for example, writes of the need that homeless mentally ill women have for individualized interventions: 'In my view, the big mistake people make in trying to help the homeless is that they expect, or hope, that one single solution will solve the problems of all of us. Generally we, the homeless, are viewed as strands on the same gray mop ... My view from the park bench, from the narrow cot in crowded shelters, from the shuffling lines at feeding stations is that we are not all alike by any means and that, in fact, the solution for one of us can spell disaster for another.'

*Some Neglected Points*

The foregoing observations reveal that, generally speaking, there is considerable concordance between the expressed service needs of patient-authors and the notions that, at least in theory, increasingly inform professional planning efforts. This should be gratifying to program planners who have apparently not, from the point of view of patient-authors, gone off into orbits that are removed from their expressed concerns.

That is the good news. At the same time, however, the patient-authored literature reveals a number of relevant notions and ideas that are, at best, rarely given credence by professional program planners. Among these are the importance of hope to patients, their need for validation and encouragement, and their wish to be more fully involved in program-planning efforts. A patient at the Rhode Island Institute of Mental Health (1984) who signs her name as Hilda expresses the need for hope in a short poem:

> I've got room for friends
> I've got room for sunshine
> I've got room for laughter
> I've got room for fortune
> I've got room for tomorrow

And the futility of having no hope is poetically documented in narrative form by Leete (1987): 'We are met by profound silence by all when we ask if we will ever be all right. Imagine our feelings of worthlessness as we are continually bounced from hospital to hospital, transferred from doctor to doctor, switched from one medication to another, and thrown into one living situation after another, making any kind of coordinated or consistent treatment impossible and only convincing us further that our situation is hopeless. The only uniform messages we get from others are that we are incapable of functioning successfully, that we cannot be independent, that we will never get well.' Thus, patient-authored writings strongly emphasize that where there is no hope there can be no improvement: that where there is no hope the patient is doomed to desolation. And although I have, in the course of my professional lifetime, reviewed many professionally authored articles on mental health program planning, I remember very few that deal with the idea of hope in any way, shape, or form.

This is true also for discussions of the role of professionals in instilling hope. The patient-authored literature is strong in stating that, in order for hope to flourish, patients must be given a chance by their caregivers. They must be engaged through encouragement and support from professionals who validate their ability to change – a sentiment simply but very forcefully expressed by Peterson (1978), a former patient who is a member of the Fountain House program in New York City: 'For me, rehabilitation is not having something done to me.'

Still another theme related to hope that is prominent in the patient-authored literature, but once again largely ignored in the professional literature, is the notion that hope is often an outgrowth of a special relationship between patient and therapist. Leighton (1988, p. 71), a former patient who is currently the director of the Family and Individual Reliance Project for the Mental Health Association of Texas, writes of a particular psychologist: 'She was more human than any of the other doctors I had seen and treated me more humanely. There was a rapport and an equality between us ... With the other doctors I had seen, I felt inferior in their presence. Of course, my ego was badly damaged by the illness. But their superior attitudes hurt me even more. This psychologist treated me like one human being helping another. For the first time, strength in me was recognized and fostered. Early in her treatment of me, she let me know I had responsibility over my own illness and wellness. She insisted that I try, something never suggested previously. Her expectations of me and the hard work she demanded on my part are the major reasons I recovered.'

Time and time again the patient-authored literature reinforces the reciprocity between establishing a special and productive therapeutic relationship, the emergence of a feeling of acceptance, the birth of hope, and the beginnings of improved functioning. Lovejoy (1984) explains that, when these came together for her, she was able to change her life 'through the help of others rather than being a passive victim, and to replace self-pity and helplessness with courage and honesty' (p. 810).

The lesson here for professionals is evident. Since their needs and characteristics differ widely, patients may possibly have a better prognosis in some other program, in some other place, or with some other clinician. Professional planners must be prepared to acknowledge this circumstance and grant flexibility in program development (Bachrach, 1989).

Patient-authors also stress in their writings – and, once again, this emphasis is generally absent from the professional literature – a strong desire to be more fully involved in their own program planning. The failure to consult patients in matters that affect their own welfare is widely perceived among patient-authors as demoralizing and dehumanizing. A patient at the Rhode Island Institute of Mental Health (1984) who signs his name as Gavin describes the hopelessness that results from his inability to control the direction of his life:

> My whole life has been
> Wrapped up in the way
> Doctors, nurses, mental attendants
> Make a discussion over
> How to live my life in the hospital
> I've been in institutions so long
> I can't make a decision
> On my own

For some patient-authors the need for personal involvement in the planning process is expressed as a desire for more mutual help and peer-support groups. Chamberlin's *On Our Own* (1978) has become a classic reference for the development of patient self-help groups. Field (1988) reports on his attendance at a conference organized for former patients: 'It's hard to describe how good it feels to be surrounded by hundreds of people who know what you're talking about. It was travelling one thousand miles only to find yourself at home.'

**Analysis and Discussion**

It is important to acknowledge that, although this analysis of patient-authored literature documents some general emphases and perhaps provides tentative direction for program planners, it also contains some serious methodological difficulties. Because the material examined can generate profound personal reactions and can lead to highly subjective conclusions, I have resisted referring to this work as a bona fide content analysis, and I have not presented my findings in a quantitative format. This, of course, makes it difficult to replicate the findings reported here and to verify their validity.

A cautionary word about the generalizability of these findings is also in order. The literature reviewed for this analysis reflects only the views of those patients or former patients who write, and there is obviously a possibility that they do not represent the majority of mentally ill individuals. On the other hand, these writings most assuredly do reflect the thinking of some current and former patients; and if we are attempting to listen to what patients have to say, we might just as well start with those who, by virtue of their writing, have indicated a willingness and an ability to share their thoughts. Accordingly, the observations made here should perhaps be understood more as hypothesis-generating statements than as definitive findings.

There is, none the less, a strong indication that attending to the patient-authored literature, which is obviously a just and humane exercise, is also a sensible thing for professionals to do, for they stand to learn much from the experience. For example, McKay (1986, p. C3) writes of her stay in a psychiatric ward: 'Drugs every few hours. Forced recreation. Scolding if you lie down too much. Nothing to do but smoke. Boredom. Everyone half-stupefied under medication. The smell of hospital everywhere.'

By contrast, life on the streets, though hardly desirable, offers some meager rewards: 'There is something to do outside [the hospital]. Something to look at. The homeless can go to their favorite corner to beg ... Once or twice, if they're lucky begging, they can go for a cup of coffee. They can hope that the next day will be different. They can make plans for themselves ... Inside an institution, there is nothing to do for yourself, for your future' (ibid.).

Statements like these suggest that homelessness for mentally ill persons more often reflects service-system deficiencies than it does an individual's abstract 'choice' to live on the streets. Indeed, an anonymous report by a patient living in Oklahoma addresses the matter of choice directly: 'Someone who has been on the streets and is homeless and jobless and who has a disability, who doesn't have a car or food or a friend, and doesn't know what to do to change their situation, is in pain. Most people would probably agree that if given a choice they would trade that level of emotional pain for some good old-fashioned physical hurt anytime. But there is no choice. If you talk to someone who has been there, they will tell you they were alone and afraid. So afraid that help doesn't look like help, but like more torture' (Anonymous, 1988).

The patient-authored literature also reveals that the mental health service system may be different things at different times to different patients; or even to the same patient at different times – a fact that service planners frequently overlook. Leighton (1988) writes: 'I'm one of the fortunate ones. I learned the hard way that what happens in the mental health system is not always good for your mental health. But sometimes it is. And for me, that's made all the difference' (p. 73).

Those in the professional community who are inclined – and often with good reason – to view the service system as a massive monolith impervious to change may take heart from these words and be motivated to assume greater flexibility in their program planning as they respond to this variability.

Perhaps, most important, however, the patient-authored literature can provide the professional planner with a heightened sense of the profoundness of patients' secondary disabilities – the vastness of their shattered hopes and terrible frustrations. Armed with this knowledge, mental health professionals may wish to call into question the very language that they employ. For example, Leighton (1988) writes: 'Being called "chronic," as I was, was killing ... It made me feel so helpless and hopeless. It made me want to give up. That's why as a mental health consumer advocate, I try to help change the terminology from "chronic" to "long-term"' (p. 66).

Many professionals, I among them, see some positive value in using the word 'chronic' and in not substituting other terminology which will probably turn out to be just as stigmatizing. They fear, moreover, that playing fast and loose with language might even have negative consequences, costing patients some of their entitlements and benefits (Bachrach, 1988). None the less, Leighton's words carry an undeniable emotional force that may move professionals to understand that their 'neutral' academic approach is really very charged for patients. From such understanding comes the possibility of change.

**Concluding Comments**

We have seen that the substantive value of patient-authored literature is considerable. The literature is replete with perspectives that are relevant to mental health program planning, and these may be advantageously exploited by the professional community.

Beyond these substantive contributions, however, lie other important, albeit less tangible, benefits. Patient-authored writings generate a heightened awareness of the complexities surrounding relevant and sensitive program planning. Services for mentally ill persons must consist of much more than prefabricated program elements selected from a menu of offerings: they must be constructed with appreciation of the needs and hopes of the individuals who are to be served.

For me the experience of reviewing the patient-authored literature has been an introduction to humility, and in that vein I conclude with a moving quotation from an article by a former patient, Bockes (1985, p. 489): 'I still have a long road ahead of me. There is much that I don't understand about schizophrenia, but I realize I am not alone in my lack of knowledge about the illness. Slowly I am learning to accept the limitations of my illness, and I feel that I am beginning to make more constructive choices than I have in the past. Life puts various limitations on each person, but within those limitations there is always the freedom to make certain choices – an insight that I find relieving as well as revealing.' The professional community stands to learn a great deal from this and other extraordinary statements that make up the literature of patient-authors.

REFERENCES

Allen, P. (1974). A consumer's view of California's mental health care system. *Psychiatric Quarterly, 48*, 1–13.

Anonymous. (1986, 18 March). I feel I am trapped inside my head, banging against its walls, trying desperately to escape. *New York Times*, p. C3.

Anonymous. (1988, Summer). Someone who has been there. *Newsletter of New Beginnings*, Elgin, OK, unpaginated.

Bachrach, L.L. (1987). *Leona Bachrach speaks: Selected speeches and lectures*. San Francisco: Jossey-Bass.

Bachrach, L.L. (1988). Defining chronic mental illness: A concept paper. *Hospital and Community Psychiatry, 39*, 383–388.

Bachrach, L.L. (1989). The legacy of model programs. *Hospital and Community Psychiatry, 40*, 234–235.

Bachrach, L.L., Talbott, J.A., & Meyerson, A.T. (1987). The chronic psychiatric patient as a 'difficult' patient: A conceptual analysis. In A.T. Meyerson (Ed.), *New directions for mental health services: Barriers to treating the chronic mentally ill*, Vol. 33 (pp. 35–50). San Francisco: Jossey-Bass.

Beeman, R. (1988, October). You're sort of trapped in this inner world in seeds of crisis. *Special Report of the Mesa-Tempe-Chandler* (Arizona) *Tribune*, 28 September–2 October, p. 4.

# Families and Mental Illness: What Have We Learned?

## FROMA WALSH

Clinical views of and approaches with families of the mentally ill have undergone important transformations over the past two decades. This essay focuses on two major paradigmatic shifts that have occurred in our thinking and practice – namely, a shift towards a biopsychosocial orientation and a shift from viewing families as pathogenic influences to involving them as valued resources and collaborators in the treatment process. These changes in our perspective are examined here as they concern the role of the family in the development, course, and treatment of serious mental illness. As well, the promising new approaches for effective long-term adaptation and the principles that guide these family-oriented intervention strategies are highlighted.

### A Biopsychosocial Systems Orientation

Historically, there has been a tendency in the field of mental health for opinion about the cause of major mental disorders to swing back and forth between the dichotomous assumptions of biological and social causality. Attempts to understand the transmission of schizophrenia, in particular, have been plagued by simplistic either/or arguments for genetic versus environmental explanations. This tendency has fostered controversy over the role of the family in the development and course of the illness and family involvement in various intervention strategies. Clinical theory and research on schizophrenia have exemplified this polarization of opinion. At one extreme are those who have argued that schizophrenia is merely a myth or a metaphor, symptomatic of the 'real' problem: the family that has caused it, or at the least, needs to maintain it to serve a function. Adherents of this view oppose any labelling of illness, as well as any diagnosis, hospitalization, or medication that, they argue, fosters a stigmatizing 'patient' identity and chronic course (Haley, 1980). At the other extreme, biological determinists have tended to rely on psychopharmocological interventions, failing to see any value in involving families in treatment.

In the early 1970s I was fortunate to participate in a research program (Walsh, 1987) led by the eminent psychiatrist Roy Grinker, Sr, who had the vision to see a biopsychosocial systems orientation as fundamental to the study and treatment of schizophrenia, borderline disorders, and other serious mental conditions. This appreciation of the importance of both nature and nurture addresses the reciprocal influences of the individual, the family, and larger social systems that occur in their ongoing interactions. This orientation guides all of my clinical thinking and my approach with seriously disturbed patients and their families. Yet, throughout clinical research and practice, despite increased awareness of the complicated, mutual influences between biological and psychosocial factors, this biopsychosocial perspective has not been well integrated into most treatment of schizophrenia and other major mental disorders.

## From Deficit to Resource Models of the Family

Assumptions about family normality and pathology, embedded in our cultural and professional belief systems, underlie all clinical theory and practice (Walsh, 1993a). Such constructions exert a powerful influence in clinical assessment of families and approaches to therapeutic intervention. Until recently, the prevalent view of the family has been pathology-based, seeking to explain a wide range of individual disorders as rooted in negative family influences. Traditionally, family assessment has been so deficit-focused that family strengths and resources have been either overlooked or misconstrued as pathogenic. In the first edition of *Normal Family Processes*, published in 1982, I remarked – only half-jokingly – that a normal family could be defined as one that had not yet been clinically assessed.

Now, a decade later, with the second edition of the volume (Walsh, 1993b), I have been greatly encouraged by a fundamental shift that has occurred in clinical theory, research, and practice towards recognition, respect, and support of family strengths. A survey of these developments follows, with particular attention paid to research advances in schizophrenia and the potential they hold for more effective intervention and family support with a range of chronic mental illnesses.

## From Schizophrenogenic Mother to Interactional View

Before the turn of the century, in the first attempt to classify mental disorders, Kraepelin posited a biological base in schizophrenia, then known as 'dementia praecox' (Walsh, 1987). But by the 1940s, with the growing influence of the psychoanalytic movement, clinicians and investigators sought to uncover a psychosocial etiology of the disorder. On the basis of theories of child development and psychopathology, it was presumed that the most serious and chronic disorders must have their origins in the earliest mother–child bonds in infancy. The term 'schizophrenogenic mother,' coined by Frieda Fromm-Reichmann (1948), referred to deficiencies in the mother's character and parenting style deemed responsible for schizophrenia in an offspring. A spate of impressionistic case-studies by clinicians – many of whom had never met the parents of their patients – posited an array of deficiencies in the supposed 'schizophrenogenic mother,' ranging from symbiotic overinvolvement, overprotectiveness, and intrusiveness, to cold, harsh, rejecting attitudes. In narrowly focusing on the mother–child dyad, scant attention was directed to other family or social variables, other than a few references to a 'peripheral father.'

Throughout much of the clinical literature, families have been portrayed as noxious and destructive environments. Mothers, because of their culturally prescribed centrality in childrearing (McGoldrick, Anderson, & Walsh, 1989), have received the harshest scrutiny and have been blamed for any and all problems in the lives of their offspring. The following excerpt from a case analysis published in a leading psychiatric journal in the 1940s is unfortunately typical of mother-blaming indictments that have persisted: 'In this paper, it has been possible to examine minutely a specific family situation. The facts speak rather boldly for themselves. The mother and wife is a domineering, aggressive, and sadistic person with no redeeming good qualities. She crushes individual initiative and independent thinking in her husband, and prevents their inception in her children. The latter, particularly, are open to no counterbalancing, healthy social forces' (Gralnick, 1943, p. 324).

The view that sees 'no redeeming good qualities' in the mother and the absence of 'counterbalancing, healthy social forces' condemns the mother as a person and blames her for, so to speak, sins of commission. The father, portrayed as weak or peripheral, is, in contrast, chastised for sins of omission – for failing to assert his culturally normative strong, dominant role in the family to counteract the mother's 'domineering' influence. Theodore Lidz, among the most prominent leaders in psychiatry, contended that such a skewed parental relationship was one of the chief family structural deficits leading to schizophrenia in offspring (Walsh, 1993b).

In the late 1950s, a new level of observation and analysis of the whole family as an interactional system developed out of contributions from general systems theory, cybernetics, and communication theories. The family-systems perspective advanced conceptualization of the family, replacing a dyadic, linear, deterministic view of family causality with the recognition of multiple, recursive influences that shape individual and family functioning (Rolland & Walsh, 1994). Still, in the early development of family-systems theory and the field of family therapy, the focus was primarily on dysfunctional family processes presumed to be implicated in the ongoing maintenance of individual symptoms, if not in their origins.

Family interaction research focused on schizophrenia. In addition to the work of the Lidz group at Yale, pioneering investigations by Gregory Bateson and his colleagues at Palo Alto led to formulation of the double-bind communication hypothesis. Projects at the National Institute of Mental Health included studies of communication deviance in parental transactions, by Lyman Wynne and Margaret Singer, and exploration of multigenerational patterns of differentiation, by Murray Bowen. As innovative as those early family-process studies were, most (like the earlier case-studies) were criticized for methodological weaknesses and lacked confirmation in more systematic investigation as psychiatric interest and funding priorities shifted to the biological bases of schizophrenia (Walsh, 1988).

More recent family studies have assumed the ongoing mutual influence of biological and environmental factors and have shifted focus from questions of origin to attempts to understand ongoing transactional processes that can influence the future course and outcome of an illness. The most promising line of inquiry has examined contributions of family communication processes and attitudes towards the patient. Lyman Wynne and his colleagues have pursued a series of carefully designed studies of family communication processes as they interact with genetic predisposition. Investigations by Brown and colleagues (Brown, Birley, & Wing, 1972) and by Vaughn and Leff (1976) have found empirical evidence linking the course of a schizophrenic disorder with certain attitudes expressed by family members, presumably reflecting ongoing transactions. Their concept of 'expressed emotion' refers to critical comments and emotional overinvolvement, identified as highly predictive of later symptomatic relapse by the patient. Findings of relapse associated with extremes of expressed emotion in spouses and other relatives besides parents suggest that current interaction is a crucial determinant of the course of the illness.

As research has broadened beyond schizophrenia to other serious and chronic disorders, some similar patterns have emerged. Patients with severe depression have been found to be highly sensitive to criticism, which predicted their relapse. Extreme expressed emotion has also been found to predict the course of anorexia nervosa, and may have an influence on the course of other serious disorders (Leff & Vaughn, 1985). By shifting focus from cause to course of an illness, and by delineating specific elements of family process that can influence that course, we can improve our ability to target family interventions in order to alter these specific patterns and to strengthen patient and family functioning.

## Towards a Family Resilience Framework

In my own studies comparing young adult schizophrenic patients with others hospitalized for other severe emotional disorders (Walsh, 1987), I was impressed by the diversity and the range of functioning among the families we interviewed. It became evident that there is no single pattern that distinguishes a so-called schizophrenogenic family or characterizes all families with a schizophrenic member. While some families show quite disturbed transactional processes, other families could be seen to function remarkably well. Clinicians err when they presume a one-to-one correlation between patient disorder and family pathology, and when they reflexively label a family by the diagnosis of a member.

Moreover, that error wrongly stigmatizes and blames families, most of whom are coping as well as possible with the seriously disordered and often life-threatening behaviour of a family member. Much of the family distress evidenced at the hospitalization of a member is not specific to schizophrenia or other particular diagnoses, but is generated by the crisis situations the family is struggling to manage. Here, a systems perspective is needed to appreciate, not only how parents influence their offspring, but also how the disturbed behaviour of a child can have a profound impact on the family, creating stress in the parents' marital interaction and all other relationships. Too often, family distress generated by the upheaval in response to a patient's disturbed, destructive, or life-threatening behaviour is misdiagnosed as family pathology and presumed to have played a causal role in the development of the disorder. In fact, the family may be coping as well as can be reasonably expected, challenged by the family member's biologically based vulnerability and the family's depleted resources over time (Walsh & Anderson, 1988).

In many cases, clinicians err in confounding family-style variance with pathology. For example, the pathologizing label 'enmeshed family' is too readily applied to families that appear to be highly cohesive. That transactional style may be normative in their cultural context, or it may be a coping strategy the family has adopted to deal with crisis. Clinicians need to be cautious not to pathologize and stereotype families by misapplication of reductionistic labels. As Lewis, Beavers, and their colleagues (1976) observed in studies of families with a wide range of functioning, 'no single thread' distinguishes healthy from dysfunctional families.

It is crucial that we appreciate the blaming and stigmatizing experiences of families who have felt prejudged and blamed in their contacts with mental health professionals, schools, or courts. We need to disengage a family's referral for intervention from assumptions that the family is the real problem and the source of the patient's problems. Rather than presenting – or implying – family causality as the rationale for family therapy, we need to emphasize the family's crucial role in caregiving and problem solving.

The very language of therapy can pathologize families. We have become more sensitive to the blame, shame, and guilt implicit in the label 'schizophrenogenic mother,' but some family therapists have pathologized families with demeaning language and pejorative assumptions about dysfunctional families, such as 'dirty games' played by 'destructive' families with a seriously disturbed member (see a critique by Anderson, 1986). The recent bandwagon effect of popular movements for survivors of dysfunctional families has contributed to widespread parent-blaming and family-pathologizing.

I am encouraged that family therapy has most recently been at the forefront in tilting away from the earlier deficit skew and power-based strategies. We are coming to recognize that successful interventions rest as much on the resources of the family as on the skills of the therapist, and that the most effective therapeutic relationships are collaborative partnerships. Rather than viewing the family as deficient, incompetent, and resistant, this new orientation views therapists in partnership with families, building on existing and potential strengths and resources.

My own clinical approach and research have evolved towards a family-resilience framework for understanding the strengths and vulnerabilities of families as they confront inevitable life challenges (Walsh, in press).

This involves a shift in perspective from family damage to family challenge. A challenge model of family resiliency corrects the tendency to think of family strengths and resources in terms of a mythologized problem-free family. Instead, we need to understand how families can survive and regenerate even in the midst of overwhelming stress, adversity, or life-altering transition.

Funding for family research, which has been almost exclusively problem-focused, should be targeted as well to efforts to identify and better understand family strengths and successful adaptation to difficult challenges. In particular, we have much to learn from families who are able to cope effectively with the challenges of serious and chronic mental illness of a family member. Further, research efforts themselves should be conducted more as collaborative partnerships with families. Organizations like the National Alliance for the Mentally Ill might well become involved in such research, which would clearly benefit distressed families.

### Principles for Family Intervention with Serious and Chronic Mental Illness

In clinical practice, we have seen a shift in attitude and attention to the need for interventions to strengthen and support families of patients with serious disorders. Nearly three decades ago the deinstitutionalization movement placed patients in the community but failed to follow through with adequate out-patient services. In psychiatry, policies of utilization review, treatment contracts, and informed consent further reduced hospital stays. Drug management, while controlling psychotic symptoms, was insufficient in maintaining independent patient functioning in the community. The expectation for families to assume the primary caregiving burden for patients over the chronic course of an illness, and family dissatisfaction with traditional psychiatric approaches that blamed and stigmatized the family, brought increased pressure from families themselves, who have organized through the National Alliance for the Mentally Ill (NAMI) and other groups to advocate for more supportive programs and community resources (Hatfield & Lefley, 1987).

These developments have led to increased recognition of the reciprocal relationship among patients, families, and other social systems. It is a misapplication of systems theory to view all problems as stemming from a dysfunctional family. Further, clinicians should be cautious not to presume that an individual's disturbed behaviour serves a function for the family. Dysfunctional family patterns that emerge when a member is in crisis may not reflect the family's prior style or optimal level of functioning; rather, they may be stress-induced. Not only do families influence individual members, but individual vulnerabilities, disturbed behaviour, and associated stresses affect the family. The availability or lack of community supports and the acceptance or stigma associated with mental illness also influence individual and family adaptation.

Over the past decade there has been a welcome shift in attention and therapeutic aims towards greater recognition and enhancement of family strengths and resources in dealing with chronic disorders. Current approaches to family intervention are grounded in a stress-diathesis model. Assessment and intervention are aimed, not at exploring past causal factors, but instead at management of a biologically based illness, viewing the family as an indispensable ally in treatment. Stress reduction and strengthening the supportive functioning of the family, along with improved patient functioning, are inseparable goals of intervention.

The importance of family involvement in treatment is being shown in studies on a range of serious and chronic mental and physical illnesses. The psychoeducational approaches have best demonstrated their effectiveness with schizophrenia, but also show promise in the treatment of other disorders. These family interventions have been found to prevent or delay relapse, reduce family stress, and improve functioning for patients and their families. In the treatment of affective disorders, phobias, and other anxiety states, behavioural therapies involving spouses as collaborators in the treatment have been shown to be superior to individual or group treatments (Gurman, Kniskern, & Pinsof, 1986).

Psychoeducational approaches to family intervention, most notably those developed by Anderson (Anderson, Reiss, & Hogarty, 1986), Goldstein (Goldstein & Kopeikin, 1981), Falloon (Falloon, Boyd, & McGill, 1984), and McFarlane (1983), have been developed to provide information, management guidelines, and social support to families in their role as caregivers over the course of a chronic mental illness in one of their members. The model is based on the assumption that the patient has a core biological deficit and that environmental stresses interact negatively with that vulnerability to produce disturbed thinking and behaviour.

The psychoeducational approaches do much to correct the blaming, causal attributions experienced by so many families of the mentally ill (Hatfield, 1987). In contrast to more traditional treatment approaches that presume the family invariably to be a pathogenic influence on the patient, psychoeducational approaches view family members as caring and vital resources in promoting the long-term adaptation of the patient and his or her effective functioning in the community. The rationale for family intervention is based on the importance of support to the family, practical information about the illness, and problem-solving assistance through predictably stressful periods that can be anticipated in the course of a serious and chronic mental illness. By identifying common challenges, families are helped to plan how to handle stresses and prevent or buffer future crises. Multi-family groups are designed to provide social support, sharing of problem-solving experiences, and reduction of stigma and isolation.

More specifically, in the Anderson model, there are five phases of intervention. First, a connecting phase establishes an alliance with families by attending in a non-critical manner to the family's needs and experiences, and to specific areas of stress in their lives. Second, a day-long survival-skills workshop provides a group of families with current empirically based knowledge about schizophrenia and its treatment, emphasizing the importance of medication compliance to avoid relapse. Concrete principles and guidelines for managing the illness are outlined and information is provided about what families can reasonably expect. Families are encouraged to set clear limits on the patient's disruptive behaviour and to shift attention and time to other members' needs and to pursuits outside the family. This need for respite and finding time and energy away from problems is perhaps the most neglected area in traditional treatment approaches. Also, more traditional family therapies held the assumption that a brief intervention and simply attending to interrupting destructive cycles of family interaction would enable families to find better solutions and function on their own. Families confronting the demands of a serious and chronic mental illness need all the help they can get to manage their situation more effectively. They have been in a position, in traditional treatments, of being damned if they do too much and if they do too little. If they restricted a patient's behaviour outside the home out of fear that he may get out of control or destructive, they were blamed for being overprotective. If they let him go out in order to maximize his sense of self-responsibility, they were accused of being neglectful. Families greatly value management guidelines and help in setting realistic expectations.

It is important to recognize the need for combined intervention strategies in the treatment of serious and chronic disorders. Long-term drug maintenance may be necessary to control the severity of symptoms and to prevent lengthy and repeated hospitalizations. For instance, family therapy in combination with drug therapy has been found to be more effective in preventing or delaying relapse in schizophrenia than either therapy used alone. The addition of patient involvement in a social-skills group yields the best results (Goldstein & Kopeikin, 1981; Anderson, Reiss, & Hogarty, 1986).

The basic principles of the psychoeducational models can be adapted to fit varied treatment settings and practice with a range of disorders (Bernheim & Lehman, 1985). McFarlane (1983) has developed a decision tree to assist clinicians in the determination and sequencing of approaches and priorities in different case situations. Family consultation, an approach advanced by Wynne, McDaniel, and Weber (1986), shares with psychoeducational approaches a responsiveness to the family's stress as caregivers, and the setting of concrete, realistic objectives in active collaboration with the family. Families with a chronically ill member who have been critical of more traditional therapeutic approaches have responded positively to the developments of these approaches.

Brief problem-solving family therapy, providing structured, focused interventions, may be useful to many families challenged by a chronic mental illness. Improved functioning and reduced stress and relational conflict can be achieved through pragmatic focus on clear, concrete, realistic objectives that can be met over several months. Once a higher level of functioning has been stabilized, gains can be sustained and set-backs averted with monthly or periodic maintenance sessions. Multi-family therapy groups and self-help groups are especially useful for sustaining care and support over the long haul of a chronic illness.

Crisis intervention should be available to families in times of acute distress, since most severe, chronic disorders involve periodic exacerbation of symptoms. Therapists must be active and provide enough structure to help temporarily overwhelmed families reorganize and gain perspective and control of threatening situations. Because patients with serious disorders, especially schizophrenia or manic episodes, may lack motivation, use poor judgment, or fail to comply with medication regimens, family collaboration is crucial to keep patients involved in treatment and to help families cope and reduce stress to manageable proportions. Without such guidance, many patients and their families rebound from one crisis to the next; achieve few gains over time; and risk emotional exhaustion, serious conflict, and relationship cut-off.

In all clinical assessment and intervention strategies, it is vital to identify and reinforce family strengths, resources, and successful coping strategies (Walsh, 1993b). In designing clinical treatment for patients and their families, intervention priorities should include:

1  reduction of the stressful impact of the chronic disorder on the family;
2  provision of information about the illness, patient abilities and limitations, and the need for psychopharmacological interventions;
3  concrete guidelines for problem solving and crisis management
   through different phases of the illness;
4  linkage to supplementary services to support the efforts of the family to
   maintain the patient in the community.

Clinicians need to be flexible in tailoring different interventions and responding to different family members, as needs arise. The work of Stein and Test (1980) documents the importance of continuity of care and community-based management over the long-term course of serious mental illness. The families of the mentally ill are our most crucial resources; we need to value their collaboration, understand their caregiving challenges, support them in our social policies and in health-care funding, and strengthen their resilience in our clinical interventions. The recent advances in our concepts and methods offer considerable hope and promise in meeting these challenges.

REFERENCES

Anderson, C. (1986). The all-too-short trip from positive to negative connotation. *Journal of Marital and Family Therapy, 12*, 351–354.
Anderson, C., Reiss, D., & Hogarty, G. (1986). *Schizophrenia and the family.* New York: Guilford.
Bernheim, K., & Lehman, A. (1985). *Working with families of the mentally ill.* New York: W.W. Norton.
Brown, G.W., Birley, J.L.T., & Wing, J.K. (1972). Influences of family life on the course of schizophrenic disorders: A replication. *British Journal of Psychiatry, 121*, 241–258.
Falloon, I., Boyd, J., & McGill, C. (1984). *Family care of schizophrenia: A problem-solving approach to the treatment of mental illness.* New York: Guilford.
Fromm-Reichmann, F. (1948). Notes on the development of treatment of schizophrenia by psychoanalytic psychotherapy. *Psychiatry, 11*, 263–273.
Goldstein, M., & Kopeikin, H. (1981). Short- and long-term effects of combining drug and family therapy. In M. Goldstein (Ed.), *New developments in interventions with families* (pp. 5–26). San Francisco: Jossey-Bass.
Gralnick, A. (1943). The Carrington family: A psychiatric and social study. *Psychiatric Quarterly, 17*, 294–326.
Gurman, A., Kniskern, D., & Pinsof, W. (1986). Research on the process and out-

come of marital and family therapy. In S. Garfield & A. Bergin (Eds.), *Handbook of psychotherapy and behavior change* (3rd ed.) (pp. 565–624). New York: John Wiley & Sons.

Haley, J. (1980). *Leaving home.* New York: McGraw-Hill.

Hatfield, A. (Ed.). (1987). *Families of the mentally ill: Meeting the challenges.* San Francisco: Jossey-Bass.

Hatfield, A., & Lefley, H. (Eds.) (1987). *Families of the mentally ill: Coping and adaptation.* New York: Guilford.

Leff, J., & Vaughn, C. (1985). *Expressed emotion in families.* New York: Guilford.

Lewis, J., Beavers, W.R., Gossett, J., & Phillips, V. (1976). *No single thread: Psychological health in family systems.* New York: Brunner/Mazel.

McFarlane, W. (1983). Multiple family therapy in schizophrenia. In W. McFarlane (Ed.), *Family therapy in schizophrenia* (pp. 141–172). New York: Guilford.

McGoldrick, M., Anderson, C., & Walsh, F. (Eds.). (1989). *Women in families.* New York: W.W. Norton.

Rolland, J., & Walsh, F. (1994). Family therapy: Systems approaches to assessment and treatment. In R.E. Hales & S. Yudofsky (Eds.), *American Psychiatric Press textbook of psychiatry* (2nd ed.) (pp. 1177–1207). Philadelphia: American Psychiatric Press.

Stein, L., & Test, M. (1980). Alternative to mental hospital treatment: Conceptual model, treatment program, and clinical evaluation. *Archives of General Psychiatry, 37,* 392–412.

Vaughn, C., & Leff, J. (1976). The measurement of expressed emotion in families of psychiatric patients. *British Journal of Social and Clinical Psychiatry, 15,* 157–175.

Walsh, F. (1987). Family relationship patterns in schizophrenia. In R.R. Grinker, Sr, & M. Harrow (Eds.), *Clinical research in schizophrenia: A multi-dimensional approach* (pp. 137–152). Springfield, IL: Thomas.

Walsh, F. (1988). New perspectives on schizophrenia and families. In F. Walsh & C. Anderson (Eds.), *Chronic disorders and the family* (pp. 19–32). New York: Haworth.

Walsh, F. (1993a). Conceptualization of normal family processes. In F. Walsh (Ed.), *Normal family processes* (2nd ed.) (pp. 3–69). New York: Guilford.

Walsh, F. (1993b). *Normal family processes* (2nd ed.). New York: Guilford.

Walsh, F. (in press). *Strengthening family resilience.* New York: Guilford.

Walsh, F., & Anderson, C. (Eds.). (1988). *Chronic disorders and the family.* New York: Haworth.

Walsh, F., & McGoldrick, M. (Eds.) (1991). *Living beyond loss.* New York: W.W. Norton.

Wynne, L.C., McDaniel, S., & Weber, T. (1986). (Eds.). *Systems consultation: A new perspective for family therapy.* New York: Guilford.

# Reconceptualizing the Relationship among Families, Mental Illness, and the Mental Health System

## JOHN TRAINOR

In the past twenty years, few areas in mental health have undergone the kind of dramatic change that has occurred in the relationship among families, mental illness, and the mental health system. The change has been complex and multidimensional. Professional attitudes have shifted from an emphasis on the negative role played by families in the etiology and maintenance of pathology to a more supportive and respectful recognition of the burdens carried by families as they care for relatives with mental illness (Atkinson, 1986). Families themselves have emerged as major players in the mental health arena by virtue of the powerful self-help and advocacy organizations they have formed. As a result of the lobbying carried out by these organizations, government has also entered the picture and is taking an increasingly active role in defining a new relationship with families. Recognizing the importance of families, governments and regulatory agencies are taking steps to ensure that families are involved in planning and service delivery (Lefley, 1989).

One result of these changes is a proliferation of different points of view. Historically, an examination of the changing role of families would have been limited to the professional perspective. This approach suited an era when the professional point of view was considered the only important one. Recent shifts in mental health policy in Canada, and the emerging power of family organizations, have changed this view and have significantly increased the role being given to families (Macnaughton, 1992). There are now at least three essential perspectives which influence the changing relationships among families, mental illness, and the mental health system: those of mental health professionals, families, and government. Each will play an important part in the years to come as families struggle to redefine their role. This essay briefly examines the evolution and development of each of these perspectives and looks at implications for the mental health system.

## The Perspective of Professionals

Professional interest in families focuses on two main areas: the part families play in theories of mental illness, and the involvement of families in clinical treatment. From the late 1940s to the 1970s, families figured prominently in theories of causation, and particular emphasis was given to the negative role played by parents. Many professionals, for example, eagerly adopted the approach of Bateson and others, which located the source of illness (particularly schizophrenia) in patterns of family interaction (Bateson et al., 1956). Schizophrenia was seen, not as an individual illness, but as an expression of problems in the family system. For Bateson and his colleagues, the person with symptoms might be overtly ill, but the family as a whole was covertly schizophrenic. It is interesting to note that Bateson's later formulations of what came to be known as 'the double-bind theory' did not actually imply the blaming of parents. Instead, Bateson saw all family members as trapped in a pathological communication situation from which they could not escape (Dell, 1980). Other authors were more specific in blaming parents for the emergence of schizophrenia, focusing not on broader patterns of communication but on the effects of parental psychological disturbance on children. Fromm-Reichmann (1948) developed the concept of the 'schizophrenogenic mother' and described how this type of personality could produce schizophrenia. Her work led to a number of conceptual and treatment approaches which emphasized parental disturbance in families as fundamental in creating and transmitting pathology (Lidz et al., 1958; Wynne, 1970).

The various theories of family causation led to the practice of either excluding families to protect the patient or restructuring them to root out the disturbance. Several authors report that these approaches often produced tragic results in families (Lefley, 1989; Hatfield & Lefley, 1987). In addition to dealing with the impact of mental illness on a loved one, family members were made to feel responsible for causing it.

In the 1970s professionals began to change their outlook. They were spurred by two parallel developments: advances in knowledge and the emergence of the families movement. In the area of knowledge, a critique emerged of Bateson and other proponents of communication theory and theories of parental pathology (Gootnick, 1973; Bernheim, 1990). No consistent empirical basis could be found for theories of family-causation and, although some authors contended that the search itself reflected a misunderstanding of the theory, the result was a gradual change in professional attitudes (Dell, 1980). Of equal or greater importance than the weakness of family causation theories was the emergence of research in expressed emotion (EE). This approach, which looked at the emotional climate in the family, avoided the etiological debate and concentrated instead on the more immediate causes of acute episodes (Leff & Vaughn, 1981). It produced both striking research results and a practical model of intervention which redefined families as partners in the management of illness, rather than as enemies (Hogarty, Anderson, & Reiss, 1987). Despite the fact that family organizations often disliked the EE perspective and considered it a new form of blaming, it had the effect of changing the approach of professionals. A final ingredient that promoted the decline of family causation theories was increasing knowledge of the biogenetic components of major mental illness (Johnson, 1989; Natale & Barron, 1994). As these physical causes were identified and became better understood, the idea of the family context as a primary etiological agent was rejected by most professionals (Malone, 1993).

The second major factor in the evolution of the professional perspective was the emergence of the families movement (Hatfield, 1982). In the past, professionals had been influenced by changes in knowledge and the particular bias of their own profession. The families movement added a new kind of political ingredient to the debate, and it soon became clear that espousing theories of familial causation carried more risk than that of being exposed as lacking familiarity with the research literature. It now included the risk of being publicly confronted, in either conference or clinical settings, by angry family members. Particularly in the United States, where the families movement was strongest, family-causation theorists and family therapists were soon in retreat.

The attitudes of professionals to families are now complex and somewhat contradictory. In a study by Castaneda and Sommer (1989), 64 per cent of professionals felt that blaming families for the mental illness of their relatives was still common or very common. None the less, 81 per cent of professionals who expressed an opinion indicated approval or strong approval of family organizations. Bernheim (1990) summed up the current clinical approach to working with families in a set of principles for collaboration. These include: viewing relatives as important members of the caregiving network; providing adequate orientation to family members; using services to help reduce family burden; and involving families in planning.

**The Perspective of Families**

Families have faced tremendous difficulties in dealing both with their ill relatives and with the service systems that are in place to provide care (Hatfield & Lefley, 1987). They have written eloquently of their experiences and have been the subject of professional research which has explored the area of burden (Potasznik & Nelson, 1984; Pomeroy & Trainor, 1991). The experiences of families, particularly in the years since deinstitutionalization, have led to profound changes in how they see themselves and in their relationships with professionals and government.

As we have seen, in the 1950s and 1960s, families were blamed by many professionals for causing mental illness. It is hard to overestimate the damage and suffering that this caused thousands of families (Lefley, 1989). Many experienced extreme stress and guilt, and often developed health problems of their own (Thurer, 1983). But, in addition to these quite natural negative reactions, some families directed their anger into organizing themselves to form a wide range of family-run associations working for change. These organized families have led the way in reconceptualizing the relationship among families, mental illness, and the mental health system.

In reaction to being blamed for mental illness, families have developed a position which completely rejects the notion of blame. Organizations like the Schizophrenia Society of Canada argue that the real cause of schizophrenia is a biochemical imbalance which is part of a purely physical illness. As a result, the society is a major proponent of medical research into the diagnosis and treatment of this underlying illness. Family organizations have naturally allied themselves with professionals who support their views, in particular, biologically oriented psychiatrists. Of greater importance, however, is the fact that family organizations now have no hesitation in adopting positions in what was previously seen as the territory of 'experts.' Families are now key players in the ongoing process of trying to understand and explain major mental illness.

Family attitudes to the mental health system have changed almost as dramatically as their attitudes towards mental illness. A number of studies suggest that families are dissatisfied with services (Grella & Grusky, 1989; Holden, 1982; Pomeroy & Trainor, 1991; Tessler, Gamache, & Fisher 1991; Petrila & Sadoff, 1992), and while this dissatisfaction may not be new, the response of families to the situation is. Organizations such as the National Alliance for the Mentally Ill have become vocal critics of how governments and professionals run mental health systems, and now expect to be consulted when planning is taking place (Lefley, 1989). They expect services to work for both consumers and families, and to take the interests of both into account.

## The Perspective of Government

The traditional role of government in mental health has focused on two areas: developing mental health policy and funding, and, to some extent, managing a system of hospital and community services. The judgment of professionals was used to guide both of these functions. The implicit assumption in the government approach to mental health care was based on the idea that professional services, whether hospital- or community-based, represented the full extent of what could be done for people with mental illness. Families had little role, if any, to play in the equation.

In the past ten years, governments have fundamentally changed their attitude towards families. A number of factors contributed to this change. Of central importance is the vastly increased role played by families since deinstitutionalization (Hatfield, 1982). This role laid the groundwork for the emergence of powerful family organizations. Lobbying carried out by these groups has been effective in changing the views of government. The previous dominance of the professional viewpoint, which influenced government because of its grounding in expert knowledge, has been partially replaced by the views of families, which influence government because of the political power of families' organizations (Pomeroy & Trainor, 1991). In addition, families have criticized governments' reliance on professionals by pointing out that our current service systems, which were developed by professionals, have often failed to meet the needs of people with serious mental illness.

Another factor in the changing attitudes of government to families is fiscal constraint. Most governments are faced with soaring health care budgets and have come to realize that families represent both the largest and the cheapest form of care for people with serious mental illness. While this attitude may be cause for concern, it is none the less real and is shaping government action.

These factors have led to the emergence of families as important players in the eyes of government. As a result, governments across Canada are now reconceptualizing their approach to families (Macnaughton, 1992). This is happening in three ways:

• Families are being seen as key players in the design and planning of mental health services.

- Family organizations are being recognized as both effective lobbyists and legitimate recipients of government resources to take action on their own behalf.
- Family organizations are being viewed as competitors for service-delivery dollars. The idea that services must be controlled by professionals is losing ground.

One outcome of this emerging recognition of families is a new role for government. Instead of simply translating professional perspectives into the components of a service system, governments must now act as arbiters in a complex field with more than one interest group. In particular, families and consumers are now demanding to be recognized and to have their interests protected. In Canada, a number of provinces are translating this new and plural reality into policy (Macnaughton, 1992). Ontario, for example, has enshrined the position of families in its vision of a reformed mental health system (Ontario Ministry of Health, 1993). Families are defined as partners, and their inclusion in all aspects of planning and operating the mental health system is now mandatory, not optional.

## Conclusion

In the past, the professional viewpoint was central to determining the relationship among families, mental illness, and the mental health system. The area is now more complex and is shaped by the multiple perspectives of families, professionals, and government. The result of this has been an increasingly proactive role by government and families at the expense of professionals. Families, driven by their experiences as caregivers, have become increasingly organized and militant. Governments, under pressure from family lobbyists and increasingly constrained budgets, have become much more interested in families as partners in providing care. Taken together, these developments have dramatically changed the landscape in mental health.

Many professionals working in the field today find this situation both difficult and challenging. They were trained in the era when the professional viewpoint determined our understanding of, and response to, mental illness. The emergence of powerful family organizations and their impact on government have required changes in this outlook. There is increasing recognition by professionals of the role played by families and the burdens they carry (Atkinson, 1986; Backer & Richardson, 1989).

Rather than blaming families, many professionals are now providing support and building therapeutic alliances.

Government, families, and professionals are all players in the mental health system. As such, they can best serve consumers, who are the most fundamental stakeholders, by working together in partnership.

REFERENCES

Atkinson, J. (1986). *Schizophrenia at home.* London: Croom Helm.

Backer, T., & Richardson, D. (1989). Building bridges: Psychologists and families of the mentally ill. *American Psychologist, 44,* 546–550.

Bateson, G., Jackson, D.D., Haley, J., & Weakland, J. (1956). Toward a theory of schizophrenia. *Behavioural Science, 1,* 251–264.

Bernheim, K.F. (1990). Principles of professional and family collaboration. *Hospital and Community Psychiatry, 41,* 1353–1355.

Castenada, D., & Sommer, R. (1989). Mental health professionals' attitudes toward the family's role in the care of the mentally ill. *Hospital and Community Psychiatry, 40,* 1195–1197.

Dell, P. (1980). Researching the family theories of schizophrenia: An exercise in epistemological confusion. *Family Process, 19,* 321–335.

Fromm-Reichmann, F. (1948). Notes on the development of treatment of schizophrenics by psychoanalytic psychotherapy. *Psychiatry, 11,* 263–273.

Gootnick, A.T. (1973). Double bind hypothesis: A conceptual and empirical review. *Journal Supplement Abstract Service Catalog of Selected Documents in Psychology, 3* (86), Manuscript 417.

Grella, C., & Grusky, O. (1989). Families of the seriously mentally ill. *Hospital and Community Psychiatry, 40,* 831–835.

Hatfield, A.B., & Lefley, H.P. (1987). *Families of the mentally ill: Coping and adaptation.* New York: Guilford.

Hatfield, A.B. (1982). Therapists and families: Worlds apart. *Hospital and Community Psychiatry, 33,* 513–519.

Hogarty, G., Anderson, C., & Reiss, D. (1987). Family psychoeducation, social skills training and medication in schizophrenia. *Psychopharmacology Bulletin, 23,* 12–13.

Holden, D.F. (1982). How families evaluate mental health professionals, resources, and effects of illness. *Schizophrenia Bulletin, 8,* 626–633.

Johnson, D.L. (1989). Schizophrenia as a brain disease: Implications for psychologists and families. *American Psychologist, 44,* 553–555.

Leff, J., & Vaughn, C. (1981). The role of maintenance therapy and relatives' expressed emotion in the relapse of schizophrenia: A two-year follow-up. *British Journal of Psychiatry, 139,* 102–114.

Lefley, H.P. (1989). Family burden and family stigma in major mental illness. *American Psychologist, 44*, 556–560.

Lidz, T., Cornelison, A., Terry, D., & Fleck, S. (1958). Intrafamilial environment of the schizophrenic patient: VI. The transmission of irrationality. *A.M.A. Archives of Neurological Psychiatry, 79*, 305–316.

Macnaughton, E. (1992). Canadian mental health policy: The emergent picture. *Canada's Mental Health, 40*(1), 3–7.

Malone, J.A. (1993). Beyond blame and shame: Families coping with long-term mental illness. In. L. Chafetz (Ed.), *New directions for mental health services: A nursing perspective on severe mental illness, 58,* 43–52. San Francisco: Jossey-Bass.

Natale, G., & Barron, C. (1994). Mothers' causal explanations for their son's schizophrenia: Relationship to depression and guilt. *Archives of Psychiatric Nursing, VIII,* 228–236.

Ontario. Ministry of Health. (1993). *Putting people first: The reform of mental health services in Ontario.* Toronto: Author.

Petrila, J.P., & Sadoff, R.L. (1992). Confidentiality and the family as caregiver. *Hospital and Community Psychiatry, 12,* 136–139.

Pomeroy, E., & Trainor, J. (1991). *Families of people with mental illness: Current dilemmas and strategies for change.* Toronto: Canadian Mental Health Association.

Potasznik, H., & Nelson, G. (1984). Stress and social support: The burden experienced by the family of a mentally ill person. *American Journal of Community Psychology, 12,* 589–607.

Tessler, R.C., Gamache, G.M., & Fisher, G.A. (1991). Patterns of contact of patients' families with mental health professionals and attitudes toward professionals. *Hospital and Community Psychiatry, 42,* 929–935.

Thurer, S.L. (1983). Deinstitutionalization and women: Where the buck stops. *Hospital and Community Psychiatry, 34,* 1162–1163.

Wynne, L. (1970). Communication disorders and the quest for relatedness in families of schizophrenics. *American Journal of Psychoanalysis, 20,* 100–114.

# Shifting Domains of Illness Management: A Model of Familial Relationships in Families with a Mentally Ill Relative

## DALE BUTTERILL AND JANE PATERSON

The role of family therapy has gradually been eroded in the treatment and understanding of families dealing with an adult member who has a serious mental illness. It has been replaced by educational programs offered by professionals (Anderson, Hogarty, & Reiss, 1980) and peer-led family groups, usually under the auspices of a family association, such as Ontario Friends of Schizophrenics. This development is viewed in the main as a positive step towards reframing the roles and needs of families and removing the stigma associated with mental illness in the family. It is linked with a non-blaming stance on the part of mental health professionals as it focuses on family needs and family capabilities rather than on pathology. For these reasons, the replacement of family-therapy models with educational programs and peer-led associations has been welcomed by families as well as by many professionals (Lefley, 1989; Ontario Friends of Schizophrenics, 1992; Canadian Mental Health Association, 1991).

This essay discusses the consequences of this development and suggests that this approach has overly narrowed the range of helping responses available to families. The reasons for disenchantment with family therapy, and the subsequent development of more 'family relevant' approaches, are examined here, as is the feasibility of reincorporating family therapy and the views of consumers into the range of interventions used by professionals who work with families of the mentally ill. A model that illustrates the specific stages that families and individuals move through during the illness and recovery process is presented. The model proposes that, to be most helpful, 'stage appropriate' interventions, which range from self-help to family therapy, must be offered.

**Disenchantment with Family Therapy**

Family therapy and, by extension, theories of family functioning have become synonymous with the causal linking of the family to the illness (Nichols, 1991; Wynne, Shields, & Sirkin, 1992). The basis for this thinking is found in the work of Lidz, Cornelison, and Fleck (1958), Fromm-Reichmann (1948), and Bateson (1960), all of whom linked the appearance of the disorder, schizophrenia, to dysfunctional communication patterns. Fromm-Reichmann attributed the development of the disorder to the problem of the 'schizophrenogenic mother' in 1948. In Bateson's early work on the double-bind, his perspective too was etiological – that is, the parental double-bind created schizophrenia in the offspring (Dell, 1980). The fact that this early work represented a major conceptual shift from individual etiological factors to social/interpersonal factors was overshadowed by concern about the damaging effects of such labelling on families themselves. Although the family-therapy field moved quickly to separate the concept of causality from the examination of family communication patterns, as in the work of Bateson (1963) and that of Haley, Jackson, and Wynne, the perception of causality has persisted (Dell, 1980).

A second problem families have with theories of family functioning is the concept that 'symptoms serve a purpose,' which implies that the family needs a problem in order to function. Families quite rightly wish to be seen as helpers and not as 'patients' (Nichols & Schwartz, 1991). In fact, Wynne points out that the notion of 'family as patient' is entirely at odds with Western cultural tradition (Wynne, Shields, & Sirkin, 1992).

Also contributing to the disenchantment with the family-therapy model is the perception that family therapists have too limited an interest in the actual illness of the family member and too great an interest in the family's transactional patterns. This standard family-therapy orientation arises out of the concept of circular causality. Circular causality was introduced by family therapists as an alternative to the predominant concept of linear causality, which they criticized for being 'falsely reductionistic.' Family therapists thought that circular causality offered a less stigmatizing approach to the person with the problem (Wynne, Shields, & Sirkin, 1992). The shift in subject from person to family, and in focus from individual dynamics to interactions among family members, led families to feel stigmatized by theories of family functioning.

To conclude, associations with causality, with the concept of symptoms serving a purpose, and with the therapist's lack of regard for illness factors have contributed to the rejection of models of family therapy by families of the seriously mentally ill.

### Towards a More Family-Relevant Approach

From the point of view of many families, therapists have missed the mark by failing to respond to the basic needs of the family, such as, for information, and by failing to acknowledge family burden/loss and the family's willingness to be part of the helping process (Hatfield, 1987; Ontario Friends of Schizophrenics, 1992; Potasznik & Nelson, 1984; Lefley, 1989; Fadden, Bebbington, & Kuipers, 1987). These perceptions, augmented by the explosion in biological research and the rise of family-led organizations (Chamberlain, Rogers, & Sneed, 1989), created the conditions for a new response to families. In a rather interesting transitional way, the psychoeducational groups that developed out of the work on expressed emotion (Leff & Vaughan, 1985; Strachan et al., 1989; Halford, Schweitzer, & Varghese, 1991) embodied aspects of perceived family-blaming associated with family therapy within a model educational framework designed to teach rather than treat. The educational approach has gone on to become the preferred mode for delivering services to families. Experience with the psychoeducational model has led some family spokespersons to criticize it for being too patient-centred, for example, in focusing on relapse and the family's role in preventing it (Hatfield & Lefley, 1987). More recent concerns have shifted to quality-of-life issues for families, such as the identification of threats to self-esteem, loss/separation, security, and integrity/optimism (Hatfield, 1990).

Hatfield believes that the most appropriate theoretical framework for understanding family response to the major threats associated with mental illness is that of coping and adaptation. This perspective removes the blame and places family turmoil/confusion within the context of a normal response to a major catastrophe. It helps professionals to work more empathically with families. When she examines the range of helping responses that she feels are appropriate for families, she identifies four needs: for education, support, consultation, and psychoeducation. Hatfield clearly favours the first two and is particularly sceptical of psychoeducation, as it 'lacks conceptual clarity' and is experienced by families as being critical. Consultation is seen as an alternative to family therapy as it is a process exclusively driven by the family's definition of the problem (Hatfield, 1987). Not unlike Hatfield, Terkelsen (1987) views the therapist's relationship to the family as similar in nature to that of an accountant, lawyer, or other professional. Regardless of what helping response is used, Hatfield urges professionals to be more pragmatic, less pathologizing, and more explicit about their biases and assumptions when working with families.

There is no doubt that Hatfield and others have provided a road map for professionals and have tuned them in to the experiences and needs of families. Similarly, the strength and role of family organizations have helped professionals to develop greater awareness of families and their concerns. While it appears that Hatfield's ideas have had an impact on the practice of professionals, the degree to which their thinking and conceptual models have been affected is not as evident. The literature currently has very few offerings on the subject of families and mental illness; for example, a recent survey of four major journals yielded less than 1 per cent of articles devoted to the subject (Continuing Care Division, Clarke Institute of Psychiatry, 1991). The authors wondered whether this finding reflects a conceptual impasse resulting from repeated reminders that families have suffered too long at the hands of family therapists and their theories, or if it is attributable to other causes. It should be noted that, in the United States, the National Alliance for the Mentally Ill succeeded in having federal National Institute of Mental Health (NIMH) funds for family therapy research cut off (Nichols, 1991), which may account, in part, for the dearth of literature.

Not only is a clear professional voice on the subject of families lacking, but the consumer voice is missing as well. While professionals are rethinking the relevance of circular causality and other concepts, consumers have been slow to respond to the frameworks put forward by Hatfield and others. The authors propose that a clearly articulated theory of family functioning would be the result of a synthesis of three important perspectives: that of the family, with those of the professional and the consumer.

*The Professional Perspective*

A central challenge in reintroducing family-therapy concepts to the field seems to be that of separating blame from the process of self-examination. One question which must be addressed is, how can professionals support the family in examining its assumptions, its patterns of interaction, and its style of communication without leaving the family feeling that it has caused the problem? Family therapy, unlike education and support, assists families in developing tools of observation that enable them to examine the impact of members' behaviours on one another.

A few leading figures are beginning to carve out a middle ground for family therapy by removing outmoded concepts and reformulating the way in which the professional establishes the relationship with the family (Wynne, Shields, & Sirkin, 1992; Walsh, 1989; Birchwood & Smith, 1990). Family therapy is beginning to be seen as one of several appropriate helping responses instead of the only one for all families at all times.

Wynne, Shields, and Sirkin (1992), writing on the subject of illness and family theory, suggest that professionals abandon the concept of circular causality. In relation to families coping with a major mental illness, they agree with family advocates that it is not appropriate to attribute cause to the larger system. They endorse the use of a biopsychosocial perspective that integrates the illness concept with behavioural and interpersonal processes. They also advocate restructuring the relationship between families and professionals by shifting the focus away from pathology and onto strengths, and expanding the role of the family therapist to that of systems consultant. Their middle-ground 'solution' challenges clinicians and families alike to widen their perspectives.

Harriett Lefley (1989) also believes there is a role for family therapy. Its relevance to families is that it allows them to deal with the emotional aspects of the problem and it accommodates the family's individual response. She cites a number of issues that might appropriately be worked on in family therapy, such as family guilt, balancing the needs of family members, and issues of dependence/independence.

Finally, in her latest book, Agnes Hatfield (1990) writes about family consultation for families who prefer a one-to-one relationship and have a problem that needs individual attention. She stresses that the process should be collaborative in nature and should take place when the family has a 'course of mental illness behind them.' She sees consultation and education as being complementary.

Hence, various authors have begun to argue that family therapy should be reincorporated into the range of helping responses. The argument is based on altering some of the original premises of family therapy and restructuring the relationship between families and professionals.

*The Consumer Perspective*

The relationship of the 'consumer' to the mental health system has also changed dramatically over the last ten years. Many of the changes parallel those of families, for example, the creation of self-help organizations, the assumption of advocacy roles, and increased power in decisions affecting treatment and incarceration. Consumers have started to demand that they be seen as people with abilities, not just diagnoses (Chamberlain, Rogers, & Sneed, 1989; Barnham & Hayward, 1991). Currently, the consumer-authored literature is expanding rapidly. It is attempting to insist that professionals become more cognizant of the patients' perspective and hopes to alter notions of illness, processes, and chronicity. This literature draws our attention to the consumer's desire to change, the need for hope, and the reciprocal processes involved in recovery. It emphasizes the significant role that others (families and professionals) play in terms of creating opportunities for growth and validating the person's ability to develop. Hope, especially, is deemed fundamental to the recovery process, and change is predicated on hope (Deegan, 1988; Barnham & Hayward, 1991; Leete, 1988).

Some professionals have taken a great interest in the subjective experiences of consumers and have tried to describe the recovery process from the consumer's perspective (Lefley, 1989; Strauss, 1989). Strauss has uncovered an interesting phase during the recovery process which he calls the 'key turning point.' He argues that this is the point at which the person with the illness separates from it and begins to take responsibility for his life. He starts to see himself in more integrated terms and as a person with a future. Hopes and dreams return, and the person assumes the role of 'active agent' by beginning to take realistic steps towards realizing goals (Strauss et al., 1985). Strauss's view of the person is not unlike Wynne's. He thinks of the person as a 'psychological being, biologically constituted and functioning within an environmental context' – in other words, people are 'biopsychosocial' entities.

Patricia Deegan (1988) eloquently describes her own recovery process and describes how the emergence of hope led her to begin to rebuild her life. She attributes her discovery of hope to her loved ones, who maintained their hope throughout her illness. She refers to it as an 'invitation' which she gradually accepted. Such studies have very real implications for the relationship among families, consumers, and professionals.

What stands out in the literature cited is the consumer's striving for recovery and the very real and active role he or she plays in the process. It also draws attention to the extremely important role the family and/or significant others play. Unfortunately, the family literature explores only the need for the family to deal with the stress induced by the illness and to adapt to its reality. Facilitating the recovery process and the need to have reciprocal family–consumer relationships are not discussed. In a national publication, *Schizophrenia: A handbook for families*, for example, no mention is made of the active role of the consumer or the importance of hope for recovery (Health and Welfare Canada, 1991). The coping-adaptation theory described by Hatfield (1987) views competence as the outcome of a successful coping-adaptation process. Members are expected to contribute to the level of their competence. However, nowhere does it refer to the individual reaching a 'turning-point,' separating from the illness and assuming responsibility.

What the literature suggests are two different views of the problem and two different agendas for the treatment setting. These differences place the clinician in the position of being asked to see the problem from the point of view of either the family or the consumer. Depending on the extent of the polarization, the clinician may find it impossible to engage the whole system. The clinicians' dilemma becomes one of how to incorporate family and consumer perspectives into a viable framework that is enriched as well by theories of family functioning.

*Model of Familial Relationship in Families with a Mentally Ill Relative*

This model, which has borrowed heavily from the professional, consumer, and family literature, attempts to integrate salient features of each into a comprehensive whole. From the professional literature come the concepts of influence and interaction – that is, families and consumers are interacting systems which exert influence over each other. The patient-authored literature adds the knowledge of the consumer-as-active-agent who responds to the hope held by significant others. The family literature informs us that families have requirements that need to be addressed and that the relationship with the professional community needs to be restructured in order for families to benefit from the contact. The authors take the view that these perspectives are complementary and can be unified by the shared goals of helping families to adapt and consumers to recover.

The model herein proposes that families and consumers require different interventions at different times. The 'difference' is governed by the stage the consumer and family are at with respect to the illness. Implicit in our understanding of the problem is the belief that the recovery process for both families and consumers includes the elements of acceptance, increasing competence with respect to the management of the illness, and moving beyond the illness. For this process to occur, a series of delicate transactions take place around the focal area of illness management. The family and consumer must decide who is responsible for what with regard to the management of the illness. In the initial stage, immediately following the first episode, the relationship between family and consumer is completely dominated by the events of the illness. Both family and consumer are reacting to its occurrence, and at this stage only the family has the resources to begin to manage it. Stage I interventions for the family are family education, peer support, and one-to-one professional support. For the consumer, such interventions are medical and psychosocial. As the consumer gains awareness, and her acceptance of the illness increases, she and the family enter Stage II. This stage is characterized by shared illness management and diminished reactivity to the effects of the illness. The family's willingness to share responsibility with the consumer is as critical here as is the consumer's willingness to assume greater responsibility. For the family there must be a perception of growing consumer competence and stability in order for them to relinquish control at this stage. Interventions for the family at Stage II are ongoing professional support, peer support, and skill teaching. For the individual, treatment consists of ongoing medical intervention, skill teaching, and illness management. Family issues are discussed with both family and consumer separately, using an educational model. At Stage III the management of the illness is organized as 'shifting domains' and moves under the aegis of the consumer, with intermittent family support on an as-needed basis. Reactivity to the illness has lessened further for both the consumer and the family. With management of the illness under the control of the consumer, the relationship between family and consumer is freer to take on characteristics more typical of the premorbid period. At this point, if there is a wish for an improvement in the quality of the relationship, family therapy might be an appropriate intervention.

The model is derived from its author's clinical experience, and the following vignette provides an example of a family and a consumer family member at the different stages of the model.

*Clinical Vignette*

Susan is a forty-three-year-old woman currently living with her boyfriend in a subsidized apartment. She works as a part-time nurse and is also actively involved in many consumer-survivor projects. She was first diagnosed with schizophrenia when she was twenty-one years old and a second-year university student. After an initial hospitalization, she left university to travel to Africa. Her parents, who at the time were devastated by the news of their daughter's illness, were very troubled by her decision to travel so far away from the treatment they believed that she desperately required. They believed that her judgment was very clouded by the residual symptoms of the illness, and they feared for her safety abroad. As they suspected, Susan did experience a relapse during her time abroad and had to be flown home and hospitalized for a lengthy period of time. She then embarked on a familiar 'revolving-door course,' with her community stays punctuated by hospitalizations. During this period, Susan's parents reported that they observed many episodes of her deteriorating condition and they also joined a family support group. They were placed in the position, experienced by many families, of attempting to convince her to seek treatment, or to remain on medication, while Susan struggled with her illness and consequent symptoms. The Stage I period lasted for several years and was extremely painful for both Susan and her family. With what appeared to be a deteriorating course, Susan and her family were faced with a recommendation for long-term in-patient treatment.

In the second stage, Susan fought this recommendation and began to take on more responsibility for her illness and her life. Also during this time, her father retired and took on some part-time work. Her parents had always wanted to travel during their retirement, and so they began to go on extended vacations. Susan then devoted herself to the completion of her teaching degree and she began to work part-time. She had begun to invest in her new life, accept her illness, and discover her personhood.

She has now chosen a treatment arrangement with which she feels confident, is involved in consumer–survivor activities, lives independently, and enjoys a long-term relationship. She may be said to be firmly ensconced in Stage III.

Her parents continue to feel very saddened by their daughter's condition; however, they generally feel grateful that Susan's life has evolved as it has. They do, however, continue to fear that Susan may relapse, and they are very watchful for signs of deterioration as the incident below will illustrate. They seem reluctant to leave the shared illness management of Stage II and enter Stage III with Susan.

This situation became apparent when Susan described to her therapist her upset over feeling that her parents tended to exclude her and her boyfriend in conversation during family gatherings. Her therapist encouraged Susan to speak to her mother about this, which Susan did. Her mother then contacted the therapist, asking if Susan was becoming ill again. Her mother was reassured that Susan was upset, not ill, and was simply trying to improve her relationship with her parents. For Susan and her family, it was extremely helpful to have her upset feelings normalized instead of pathologized, and to have clarified that Susan was the one in charge of managing her illness.

This shift from illness management to family interactional issues is critical if the ill relative is to reach his or her full recovery potential. Susan now talks about her desire to enjoy her relationship with her parents and her wish to contribute to their happiness in their retirement.

Joseph Walsh (1989) points out that most of the literature on the clinical treatment of schizophrenia focuses on medication and case management rather than on developmental and relationship issues. While we do not minimize the importance of these treatments, we would argue that important relationship issues and their ensuing dynamics also need to be addressed.

The model 'shifting domains of illness management' is in the very early stages of development. It has been heavily influenced by the family, the consumer, and the professional literatures. It is intended to be a conceptual tool for all parties and does not presume to have all the answers. Its usefulness may lie in being able to identify family systems that are at different stages in the recovery process and to propose stage-appropriate interventions that will assist the entire system to realize its full potential.

REFERENCES

Anderson, C., Hogarty, G., & Reiss, D. (1980). Family treatment of adult schizophrenic patients: A psychoeducational approach. *Schizophrenia Bulletin, 6,* 400–505.

Barnham, P., & Hayward, R. (1991). *Illness and personhood.* London: Tavistock/ Routledge.

Bateson, G. (1960). Minimal requirements for a theory of schizophrenia. *Archives of General Psychiatry, 2,* 477–491.

Bateson, G. (1963). A note on the double bind. *Family Process, 2,* 154–161.

Birchwood, M., & Smith, J. (1990). Relatives and patients as partners in the management of schizophrenia. *Psychosocial Rehabilitation Journal, 13* (3), 27–30.

Canadian Mental Health Association. (1991). *Families of people with mental illness, current dilemmas and strategies for change.* Toronto: Author.

Chamberlain, J., Rogers, J., & Sneed, C. S. (1989). Consumers, families and community support systems. *Psychosocial Rehabilitation Journal, 12* (3), 93–106.

Continuing Care Division, Clarke Institute of Psychiatry. (1991). *Family literature survey*, unpublished. Toronto.

Deegan, P. (1988). Recovery: The lived experience of rehabilitation. *Psychosocial Rehabilitation Journal, 2* (4), 11–19.

Dell, P.F. (1980). Researching the family theories of schizophrenia: An exercise in epistemological confusion. *Family Process, 19* (4), 321–335.

Fadden, G., Bebbington, P., & Kuipers, L. (1987). The burden of care: The impact of functional psychiatric illness on the patient's family. *British Journal of Psychiatry, 150,* 285–292.

Fromm-Reichmann, F. (1948). Notes on the development and treatment of schizophrenics by psychoanalytic psychotherapy. *Psychiatry, 11,* 263–273.

Halford, K., Schweitzer, R., & Varghese, F. (1991). Effects of family environment on negative symptoms and quality of life of psychotic patients. *Hospital and Community Psychiatry, 42,* 1241–1247.

Hatfield, A. (1987). Families as caregivers: A historical perspective. In A. Hatfield & H. Lefley (Eds.), *Families of the mentally ill: Coping and adaptation* (pp. 3–29). New York: Guilford.

Hatfield, A. (1990). *Family education and mental illness.* New York: Guilford.

Hatfield, A., & Lefley, H. (Eds). (1987). *Families of the mentally ill: Coping and adaptation.* New York: Guilford.

Health and Welfare Canada. (1991). *Schizophrenia: A handbook for families.* Ottawa: Author

Leete, E. (1988). A consumer perspective on psychosocial treatment. *Psychosocial Rehabilitation Journal, 12* (2), 46–52.

Leff, J.P., & Vaughan, C. (1985). *Expressed emotion in families: Its significance for mental illness.* New York: Guilford.

Lefley, H. (1989). Family burden and family stigma in major mental illness. *American Psychologist, 44,* 556–560.

Lidz, T., Cornelison, A., & Fleck, S. (1958). Intrafamilial environment of the schizophrenic patient: The transmission of irrationality. *Archives of Neurological Psychiatry, 79,* 305–316.

Nichols, M. (1991). *Family therapy: Concepts and methods.* Boston: Allyn and Bacon.

Ontario Friends of Schizophrenics. (1992, Summer). *Ontario Friends of Schizophrenics advocate.* Toronto: Author.

Potasznick, H., & Nelson, G. (1984). Stress and social support: The burden experienced by the family of a mentally ill person. *American Journal of Community Psychology, 12,* 589–607.

Strachan, A., Feingold, D., Goldstein, M., Miklowitz, D., & Nuechterlein, K. (1989). Is expressed emotion an index of a transaction process? III: Patients coping style. *Family Process, 28,* 169–181.

Strauss, J. (1989). Subjective experiences of schizophrenia: Toward a new dynamic psychiatry – II. *Schizophrenia Bulletin, 15*, 179–187.

Strauss, J., Harez, H., Lieberman, P., & Harding, C. (1985). The course of psychiatric disorder, III: Longitudinal principles. *American Journal of Psychiatry, 142*, 289–296.

Terkelsen, K. (1987). The evolution of family response to mental illness through time. In A. Hatfield & H. Lefley (Eds.), *Families of the mentally ill: Coping and adaptation* (pp. 151–166). New York: Guilford.

Walsh, J. (1989). Engaging the family of the schizophrenic client. *Social Casework: The Journal of Contemporary Social Work* (February), 106–113.

Wynne, L., Shields, C., & Sirkin, M.E. (1992). Illness, family theory and family therapy: Conceptual issues. *Family Process, 31*, 3–18.

# Out of the Ashes of Mental Illness ... A New Life

## AGNES B. HATFIELD

Considerable attention has been given in the past decade to helping professionals in the field of mental health care to better understand the family dilemma that emerges when mental illness strikes a loved one (Hatfield & Lefley, 1987; Lefley & Johnson, 1990; Marsh, 1992; Walsh, 1985; Wasow, 1982; Vine, 1982). Numerous programs have been developed to help families cope with a great array of daily problems (see, for example, Anderson, Reiss, & Hogarty, 1986; Bernheim & Lehman, 1985; Falloon, Boyd, & McGill, 1984; Hatfield, 1990; Woolis, 1992).

Educational programs for families are now widespread across the country, and most families have access to information about the nature of mental illness and an opportunity to learn management skills. The National Alliance for the Mentally Ill (NAMI) has been a powerful voice for families in making their needs known. While some families continue to suffer serious disruptions in their lives, many manage to achieve some degree of family stability. But achieving stability does not mean the end of painful issues and problems. New needs emerge when the chaos and confusion die down and family members begin to reflect upon the tragedy of their lives, the damage done to relationships, and the need to make some kind of meaning from it all.

The family faces a double tragedy if a healing process does not occur, and family relationships continue to be strained and no sense of family unity survives. The focus of family education programs is usually on survival in the here and now, but attention must also be given to the longer range issues of healing and coming to terms with the devastation.

### The Destructive Forces in Mental Illness

The destructive forces in mental illness are legion and it is surprising that families manage to survive them. Whether the onset of illness was sudden or insidious, the consequences for other members can be disastrous. My purpose here is to identify some of these potentially negative effects of mental illness and suggest ways that damage might be minimized so that growth and affirmation of life are still possible.

*Sense of Loss*

Mentally ill people lose temporarily, or permanently, many of the personality characteristics by which their relatives identify them. The changes in the person can be profound. It is as though the family has lost the person they once knew and now have a stranger in their midst. Their grief may be profound, but mourning is never complete, as it is in the case of a death, because the person continues to live, but significantly changed.

Families remember the dreams they once had, now shattered, for their relative's roles and accomplishments. Terkelsen (1987) notes that, unlike professionals who have known these individuals only in their disabled state, families knew them as well as persons full of hope and promise, and the contrast between then and now is deeply distressing. One mother wrote: It came as an utter and unbelievable surprise. We are all grieving now. We have watched a young life that was eager, healthy, attractive, with intelligence, humour, and incisive sensitivity into human relationships, waste away, without friends (when there were so many in the first twenty years), unable to stand any stress, being self conscious and terrified and almost never free from voices assailing him and sounds that he cannot bear' (Terkelsen, 1987, p. 137).

Emotional states aroused by the loss of a loved one include pain, yearning, sorrow, anguish, dejection, sadness, fear, anxiety, nervousness, agitation, panic, disbelief, denial, shock, emptiness, and lack of feeling (Schoenberg et al., 1970). Profound loss is an assault on our sense of fairness. Families who lose a relative to mental illness ask: Why did this happen to my son or daughter? What did we do to deserve this punishment? How could a just God let this happen to us? (Stearns, 1984).

Families may feel angry at those who do not understand their pain and seem so secure, safe, and distant. There is risk of bitterness, resentment, or envy towards those with healthy offspring able to lead successful lives. There may be a relentless search to find meaning in what seems to be so inexplicable, and this may lead to questions of etiology and self-blame. Family members may begin to feel extremely vulnerable. If something so disastrous can happen so suddenly and without warning, who knows what will happen next? Are any of their loved ones safe?

While we have culturally provided customs and rituals for easing the pain of those who have lost someone through death, there is little institutionalized support or practice that eases the pain of those suffering loss through mental illness (Hatfield & Lefley, 1987). Psychological theory has not been particularly relevant to supporting people faced with such existential questions of loss and deprivation (Schoenberg et al., 1970). Practitioners are on their own and, in order to be helpful, must call upon whatever personal resources and life experiences they have. Schulman (1976) says it is important not to pathologize the stressful emotions that people are undergoing and not to expect that there is an explanation for everything.

Perhaps one of the most useful books on the subject of personal loss is one written by Ann Kaiser Stearns, called *Living through personal crisis* (1984). In it she says, 'Our loses change us and change the course of our lives. It is not that one can never be happy following an experience of loss. The reality is simply that one can never again be the same' (p. 26).

Terrible events can precipitate growth, Schulman (1976) wrote in his book on coping with tragedy. People may develop a true vision of what counts, a more mature re-evaluation of their lives. They can develop a resolution of their loss so as to avoid feelings of jealousy and resentment. Joy and happiness are possible again as one realizes that going on with life does not mean abandoning the relative with mental illness. Resolution of feelings of guilt leads to inner calm.

In his discussion of chronic illness, Schulman (1976) says it is important not to view the struggle as a senseless tragedy leading to inexorable defeat, but to explore it as a creative challenge for those involved in it. Somehow out of the ashes of pain and despair may come new meaning and a way of life that can encompass the new reality. Professionals must find ways to help this process along.

*The Patient as Victim*

Because mental illness is so devastating to the individual, families may come to view their relatives as helpless victims who can do little to influence the course of their lives. They may expect little, and tolerate all misbehaviours as symptoms of the illness, while becoming increasingly resentful of the need to accommodate their lives constantly to the demands of the ill member.

It is not surprising that many people with mental illnesses assume a victim mentality, which prevents them from taking any responsibility for their own lives. Undergoing severe psychotic disturbance often means feeling oneself to be at the mercy of terrifying forces over which one has no control. As Estroff (1989) has noted, schizophrenia, in particular, seems to be an 'I am' phenomenon. Volition, self-control, and will-power seem to disappear, and patients begin to feel that they *are* their illnesses. They feel that they have lost control over their lives and are inexorably at the mercy of strange internal and external forces.

Long periods of being a patient depending on the ministrations of others may reinforce the sense of helplessness and the feeling of control by others. Other family members sympathize with the pain and struggle, and avoid expecting too much or demanding accountability. As a consequence, patients may tend to go through life expecting the rest of the world to adapt to their needs, never realizing they have obligations to others as well.

While parents often have considerable reserves of tolerance of their offsprings' self-centredness, siblings and children of mentally ill parents may expect more, and may feel resentful and rejecting when those expectations are not met. In order that family life be harmonious, attention must be given to helping the ill member learn to become a contributing member.

While classes and workshops train families to understand and care for their ill relative, similar efforts to teach the relative to understand how his behaviours affect the rest of the family are lacking. There is little evidence in the psychosocial rehabilitation literature that this matter has been considered. While attention is given to helping these individuals get along with peers, public servants, and employers, little training is offered on ways to get along with and be a contributing member of a family. This is unfortunate, when the family is recognized as a most important part of the support system. Support systems may be tenuous when obligations are totally unidirectional. Whereas parents may continue their support without reciprocity, siblings are unlikely to do so.

Parents face a creative challenge in finding ways in which a son or daughter who is mentally ill can be a contributing member. People with mental illnesses need to learn how their behaviours affect others and how to modify those behaviours to ensure the comfort of others. They need to learn ways to meet needs of other members of the family and ways of participating in family rituals, gift giving, and the like. To do less is to let the person with mental illness succumb to a perpetual-patient role.

*Volatile Behaviour*

Repeated acts of violence resulting in verbal attacks, assaultiveness, and destruction of property take a terrible toll on the family's ability to pull itself together. Relatives with mental illness may direct their hostility towards others because of jealousy, hypersensitivity to criticism, or perceived obstruction to their desires (Lefley, 1987).

The frequency with which family members suffer assault by their ill members has not been widely studied. However, Swan and Levitt (1986) studied 1,156 members of the National Alliance for the Mentally Ill (NAMI) and found that more than one-third of their respondents reported that their relative was assaultive or destructive in the home, either sometimes or often. Many families, though never assaulted, lived in fear of their relative and took self-protective measures to avoid injury.

Other family members may also be anxious about their own possible loss of control. Some mentally ill individuals can be so manipulative, hostile, argumentative, and provocative that even the most controlled persons feel that they could strike out in fear or anger (Hatfield, 1990). Under highly chaotic conditions it is likely that most members have said or done things that they have later regretted. It is a major challenge for many families to heal the wounds that might have occurred in very troubling times.

The focus must be on prevention of violence whenever possible. Families need considerable help with this, and practitioners must be ready to offer practical steps. They must understand that managing volatile behaviour in the home is much more difficult than in institutional settings. Since situational factors play a crucial role, it is important that families understand the kinds of situations that give rise to violence (Hatfield, 1990).

Even though families become adept at preventive measures, acts of aggression might occur. No violent act should be ignored, denied, or excused on the basis of mental illness. All forms of violence must be considered serious, and attention must be given to helping the perpetrator control his or her impulses. Attention must also be given to the aftermath of an attack and the devastating consequences on family feelings and relationships. The hurt is likely to continue until some kind of healing process sets in. Former NAMI president Don Richardson (1990) shares this experience of dealing with his feelings when his son assaults and seriously injures another family member: 'Without forgiveness, life is an endless cycle of rancor, hatred, and anger. I don't want to spend the rest of my

life governed by resentment and retaliation, especially toward my youngest son. I am reaching the point where I can acknowledge that this tragedy has wounded everyone in the family and now the healing process
includes forgiveness and understanding that our son's action was caused
by serious mental illness, and not because he is "evil" or "bad"' (p. 41).

*The Risk of Family Burn-out*

Even though the majority of families never experience the trauma of a
serious assault from a family member, the day-to-day managing of stressful events can take its toll when a family member serves as caregiver over
time. Some family members may choose to opt out of further involvement because they are discouraged and exhausted. Practitioners often
ask why some consumers seem to have no interested family support system. There may be many reasons, but sheer exhaustion is often one of
them.

Since there is no adequate substitute for the family as a support system,
and people with mental illness have great difficulty developing support
systems of their own, protecting the family from burn-out should be given
high priority. It is all too easy when resources are scarce to leave as much
responsibility for care to the family as long as possible, with little concern
for potential burn-out and damage to relationships over time. This is
short-sighted, for it is the consumer who suffers when families disengage
to avoid further burn-out.

## Reintegration of the Family and Role Adjustment

If the family is to survive as a unit, many adjustments must be made over
time, in various family members' roles, in apportioning responsibility in
the household, in altering social and leisure-time activities, and in finding
new ways to meet the diverse needs of all family members. Families face
difficult moral and ethical choices as they search for the right balance
between the imperatives of their ill member's care and treatment, and
the needs of other children in the family, elderly parents, and the like. It
is important that providers understand that many other demands and
stressors must be dealt with in addition to a family member's mental illness (Hatfield, 1990).

There is no single best way for families to reorganize and adapt to meet
the demands imposed by mental illness. Professionals who have strong
preconceived conceptions of how all families should function may do

more harm than good. The words of Kazak and Marvin (1988) in regard to parents of handicapped children may be instructive here. They say that 'successful adaptive functioning in families with handicapped children has not received sufficient attention. In their well-intentioned efforts to document areas of difficulty in families with handicapped children, researchers have sometimes neglected to describe ways in which differences may indicate successful family functioning within a different but not deviant family structure' (pp. 667–668). In the past, many family interventions were narrowly conceived without regard for the wide range of cultural differences in this country, and were laden with personal values as to how 'normal' families should behave (Hatfield, 1990). Many families labelled 'dysfunctional' may be merely different, and not deviant in any pathological sense.

## Conclusions

Stearns (1984) calls the last chapter of her book 'From Out of the Ashes ... New Life'. These words best express the hope for families. As Stearns has pointed out, life can never be the same again for families caring for a relative with mental illness, but happiness is possible. We can, she says, learn from our pain in such a way that our learning becomes useful to ourselves and others.

As Kushner (1981) says in his book *When bad things happen to good people*, it becomes necessary to put the past behind and cease asking the futile question 'Why did this happen to me?' Stearns (1984) sees a new kind of wisdom emerging when families can accept life as it is. 'Life as it actually is,' she says, 'though imperfect and vastly complicated with sorrow, is richer than life that is idealized' (p. 32).

Achieving this kind of wisdom is a starting-point. What must follow is the creation of a new structure and pattern to life that permits the greatest possible growth for all members of the family. As I have pointed out, the challenges are many: grieving the keen sense of loss of a loved one; healing the hurts of destructive behaviours; overcoming the identity of victimization; and just generally surviving the daily hassles that destroy morale and lead to burn-out among caregivers, to name a few.

If professionals are dedicated to preserving the family both for its own sake and because the family is vital as a support system for its ill relative, they must take a longer view of the decisions that are made and consider how they may affect the survival of the family as a supportive unit. Many family interventions at this time have a single-minded goal of helping families to create environments that are good for the ill person, with little regard for the well-being of the total family. Professionals need to take a more holistic view and be prepared to help families with the practical aspects of coping and the deeply troubling existential questions.

REFERENCES

Anderson, D., Reiss, D., & Hogarty, G. (1986). *Schizophrenia and the family*. New York: Guilford.

Bernheim, K., & Lehman, A. (1985). *Working with families of the mentally ill*. New York: W.W. Norton.

Estroff, S. (1989). Self, identity, and subjective experiences of schizophrenia: In search of the subject. *Schizophrenia Bulletin, 15*, 189–196.

Falloon, I., Boyd, J., & McGill, C. (1984). *Family care of schizophrenia*. New York: Guilford.

Hatfield, A. (1990). *Family education in mental illness*. New York: Guilford.

Hatfield, A., & Lefley, H. (Eds). (1987). *Families of the mentally ill: Coping and adaptation*. New York: Guilford.

Kazak, A., & Marvin, R. (1988). Differences, difficulties, and adaptation: Stress and social networks in families with a handicapped child. *Family Relations, 33*, 67–78.

Kushner, H. (1981). *When bad things happen to good people*. New York: Schocken Books.

Lefley, H. (1987). Behavioral manifestations of mental illness. In A. Hatfield & H. Lefley (Eds.), *Families of the mentally ill: Coping and adaptation* (pp. 107–127). New York: Guilford.

Lefley, H., & Johnson, D. (1990). *Families as allies in treatment of the mentally ill*. Washington, DC: American Psychiatric Press.

Marsh, D. (1992). *Families and mental illness*. New York: Praeger.

Richardson, D. (1990). Dangerousness and forgiveness. *Journal of the California Alliance for the Mentally Ill , 2*, 4–5.

Schoenberg, D., Carr, A., Peretz, D., & Kutschner, A. (1970). *Loss and grief*. New York: Columbia University Press.

Schulman, J. (1976). *Coping with tragedy: Successfully facing the problem of a seriously ill child*. Chicago: Follett.

Stearns, A. (1984). *Living through personal crisis*. Chicago: Thomas Moore.

Swan, R., & Levitt, M. (1986). *Patterns of adjustment to violence to families of the mentally ill*. New Orleans: Elizabeth Wisna Research Center, Tulane School of Social Work.

Terkelsen, K. (1987). The meaning of mental illness to the family. In A. Hatfield

& H. Lefley (Eds.), *Families of the mentally ill: Coping and adaptation* (pp. 151–166). New York: Guilford.

Vine, P. (1982). *Families in pain: Children, spouses, and parents speak out.* Westminster, MD: Pantheon.

Walsh, M. (1985). *Schizophrenia: Straight talk for families.* New York: Morrow.

Wasow, M. (1982). *Coping with schizophrenia: A survival manual.* Palo Alto, CA: Science & Behavior.

Woolis, R. (1992). *When someone you love has a mental illness: A handbook for families, friends and caregivers.* New York: Putnam.

# From 'Mad' to 'Bad': Helping Families Cope with Mental Illness and the Criminal Justice System

## MARLENE SWIRSKY

When Tom S. refused to continue taking his medication, his parents feared the outcome. Sure enough, within several days his behaviour began to change. He accused his parents of trying to poison him, and eventually attacked his father with a baseball bat. Frantic – and not knowing where else to turn – his parents reluctantly called the police, expecting that Tom would be taken for psychiatric treatment. At the hospital, the attending psychiatrist decided there were insufficient grounds for involuntary committal; the police, in turn, charged Tom with assault and incarcerated him, pending a psychiatric assessment.

Thus began one family's experience with the confusing and often frightening cycle of going to hospital, to jail, to court, and back again. While grateful that their son would be receiving help, Mr and Mrs S. were caught between two systems and were unprepared and uninformed regarding the type of care Tom would receive. Families in this position need help to understand the mental health and criminal justice systems and the interface between the two. Each operates under different government mandates and has different goals, but both may concurrently serve the same mentally ill offender. This situation can produce gaps in the continuity of care and/or duplication of services.

There is little documentation about the prevalence, diagnosis, functional disability, and course of mental illness among inmates in municipal, provincial, or federal institutions (Jemelka, Trupin, & Chiles, 1989; Reeder & Meldman, 1991). However, since the era of deinstitutionalization, the number of mentally ill offenders seems to have risen (Teplin, 1984; Borzecki & Wormith, 1985). The reasons for this are complex and not readily explained. It has been argued, for example, that one contributory factor has been the change in civil commitment legislation (Steadman, McCarty, & Morrissey, 1989). Mentally ill persons do not necessarily commit more crimes, but they may be arrested more frequently because of extra-legal issues (Teplin, 1986).

This essay examines the experience of families with a relative who has been ordered for a pretrial assessment. It highlights the assistance that is required and describes the clinical issues and program alternatives that are available. The population herein represents many of the chronic mentally ill in-patients who are assessed at the Metropolitan Toronto Forensic Service (METFORS) on a Warrant of Remand ordered by a provincial criminal court judge. METFORS is a unit of the Forensic Division, Clarke Institute of Psychiatry, Toronto, Ontario.

**Families and Mental Illness**

Little has been written about the family's experiences after a mentally ill relative has become incarcerated. Many have been victims of violence (Isaac & Armat, 1990), have failed in their attempts at commitment (McFarland et al., 1989), and have been forced to have their relative arrested to get the assistance they require. These same families are encouraged to go to court to testify about the dangerous aspects of their relative's behaviour. This creates an impossible dilemma for most: if testimony is given, there is significant risk that the person with the mental illness will be incarcerated rather than transferred to a psychiatric treatment setting. And while behaviour can be contained and medications reinstated in jail, it is clearly a lessthan optimal venue for those with acute psychiatric illnesses. Incarceration may offer medical stabilization, but it fails to address the complex psychosocial needs of the mentally ill offender and his or her family.

The literature on the family's role as caregiver for a chronic mentally ill relative provides relevant information about the impact of illness on significant others. The emotional consequences have been well documented. Families experience chronic emotional distress from the episodic disruptions caused by the illness. This, in turn, leaves them feeling guilty, angry, depressed, and frustrated (Hatfield, 1987a). They do not understand psychiatric symptomatology or the effects of psychotropic medications, and have endless questions about course and outcome. Families need information about mental illness and also assistance to adopt realistic expectations for their relative. As well, they need the opportunity to verbalize ambivalent feelings about their caregiving role and to obtain assistance during times of crisis. Feelings of guilt can be heightened for those who are forced to make self-protective decisions which can be misconstrued as rejection by the patient (Lefley, 1987). Thus, families have distinct needs that require both respect and attention. These burdens appear to increase exponentially for parents who are forced to cope with and need to understand both the mental health and the criminal justice system.

## Mental Illness and the Criminal Justice System

It appears that entrance into the criminal justice system is swift, and once individuals with psychiatric diagnoses have a criminal record, return to the mental health system for treatment becomes more difficult (Whitmer, 1980; Teplin, 1984; Borzecki & Wormith, 1985; Brennon et al., 1986). These mentally ill offenders are 'forfeited' because mental health professionals regard them as difficult to treat (Whitmer, 1980). Typically, these patients forget appointments, discontinue prescribed medication, deny they have a mental illness, and self-medicate with alcohol or street drugs. They often become angry, paranoid, and even threatening when assistance is offered. This group tends to drift away from services that were organized to help, and come to society's attention only when they break the law in the context of another psychotic decompensation (Whitmer, 1980). These patients are often too disorganized to be effectively antisocial and too antisocial to connect with the mental health system (Travis & Protter, 1982).

The labels 'mad,' for the mentally ill, and 'bad,' for the deviant, were used first by the criminal justice system. The relationship between these two concepts remains controversial. Antecedents of antisocial behaviours are not entirely understood. Early familial experience, underlying personality structure, and mental illness can all be contributing factors. Given this uncertainty, opinions differ with respect to patients' rights and the role of the clinician as the agent of the offender/patient, society, or the court (Cavanaugh, Wasyliw, & Rogers, 1990). Attempting to serve all three, with their often competing demands, can be complicated. Clinicians are faced with a situation in which they must balance the needs and respect the rights of all parties involved.

Families often feel guilty about being put in the position of having to testify against a son or daughter, and are often disappointed and angry that their problems are not always resolved. Clinical experience has demonstrated that each family member has a unique response to this traumatic event. These responses seem to be influenced by such factors as life-cycle stage, financial situation, and the emotional and instrumental support received from other family members. Each person is also influenced by his or her own perception of the incidents leading to the charge, knowledge of mental illness and criminal justice proceedings, and previous and current relationship with the offending relative. Families want to know how they can help their adult children who are ambivalent about psychiatric treatment. Perhaps one of the greatest problems is their relative's lack of insight or awareness of illness. After all, the person's need for medication and rehabilitation is so obvious to everyone else! Although families are relieved when a psychiatric assessment is ordered, frustration can mount to the point of being intolerable if, and when, a person refuses medication. Unfortunately, families often mistakenly assume that treatment is an implicit part of an order for a psychiatric assessment. However, in reality, a court-ordered assessment is a referral to determine the presence of mental illness and fitness to stand trial and/or the criminal responsibility of the offender.

After an assessment is completed, patients are returned to court. Here, they often face a number of remands. This situation can occur for many reasons, for example, the need to schedule a fitness hearing. If and when this happens, the mentally ill offender is detained in jail until the case is heard. For families, the fear of decompensation is great. They worry that their relative will not get the help required. Despite previous episodes of aggression and violence, the person is seen by the family as mentally ill, not criminal. Thus, families feel victimized by a system that cannot guarantee treatment. Paradoxically, patients often feel cheated and imposed upon because they have been incarcerated against their will.

*Case History*

Brian, age thirty-two, broke a window to enter his parents' home while they were on vacation. The neighbours called the police, who found him sleeping in the bathtub. They charged him with 'Breaking and Entering with Intent' and 'Unlawfully in Dwelling.'

Brian had a twelve-year history of schizophrenia. Prior to becoming ill, he had no criminal record. He had lived at home sporadically during the previous ten years, a period in which episodic assaults on his father occurred. He had been charged and placed on probation, and then lived mostly in hostels or motels. He phoned his mother and saw her occasionally, but his parents did not really know where he lived or how he spent his time. They knew he had been hospitalized on several occasions and that he would improve with medication, but would discontinue it upon discharge and gradually deteriorate.

Brian's father wanted no direct contact with his son but had called the Crown Attorney to suggest the psychiatric assessment. The judge ordered a thirty-day assessment at METFORS, and Brian was escorted to the medium-security facility by correctional officers.

Brian initially refused consent to talk to his parents, but as he stabilized on the in-patient assessment unit, he became more cooperative. His mother thought he had broken into their house because he was desperate and had no place to stay. His father said, 'Eleven years of chaos is enough,' but wanted his son rehabilitated, rather than incarcerated.

Brian agreed with his parents' opinion that he needed help to manage money, and to obtain supervised accommodation and psychiatric treatment. Discharge arrangements included a referral to welfare, the Public Trustee, a licensed boarding-home, and a case-management program. A letter was sent to the welfare office to verify the dates of incarceration and provide him with identification. Brian was released from custody, and his mother felt a renewed motivation to help him.

**Family Needs**

At METFORS, some parents prefer to talk about the patient's problems and object to questions about other family members. They want to eliminate the burden for the others. Also, recalling past episodes of the patient's abuse can be painful and emotionally overwhelming. An assault by a family member is never forgotten, especially by the victim. When one is taking a patient and family history, one must determine whether the exacerbation of the patient's symptoms and hospital admissions coincided with his or her aggressive behaviour. Obtaining details about substance abuse, family psychiatric history, and/or previous problems with the law is necessary. Additionally, the pattern of family roles and relationships, particularly with whom the patient usually argues and whom he considers helpful, is also significant.

It is important to give families the opportunity to discuss the overwhelming feelings of sadness, guilt, and anger these topics generate. Most challenging is the need to balance this respectfully with the simultaneous collection of information needed to formulate a diagnosis and describe patterns of aggression. 'Joining' with families and providing information can alleviate some of their stress. They do want to be involved and updated about issues such as medication, and assessment and treatment. It appears that having information about these issues and about what can be expected to take place at court gives some control to families who are otherwise faced with chaos. Advocating for a disposition to a hospital rather than jail can provide families with a sense of empowerment. Even if an order for hospitalization is not obtained, parents can and should be involved in the discharge planning process. They should be considered active treatment team members with valid rights and opinions. Families need help to cope with the vicissitudes of the court because it is not always easy to predict whether the next proceeding will be a remand in custody, bail hearing, trial, or sentence. The implications of these possible dispositions require clarification for all involved.

## Clinical Dilemmas

### Confidentiality

A basic tenet for professionals is to respect and maintain the confidentiality of the person they are serving. Forensic assessments by nature are not confidential because information shared can be provided to the court. Both patients and families must be advised that this is the case before pertinent issues are explored. However, one is left struggling with several important questions. For example, when a mentally ill person is in custody and has been ordered for a psychiatric assessment, should he or she have the right to deny access to a person who could provide collateral information or should information be provided to families without the patient's consent, even if the person has been deemed incompetent?

Several client systems must be engaged simultaneously: the patient, the family, the team, and the court. They often have opposing interests and competing demands. While a patient's right to privacy must be respected, this can be unfair to families who are left to 'pick up the pieces' after their relative is released. Additionally patients are motivated to find ways to obtain early release. This often means denying or minimizing symptoms or threatening behaviours, and preventing the use of contradictory evidence from others who are involved. An unfortunate consequence is that mentally ill offenders do not receive the treatment they require and are often released into the community until they decompensate and re offend. These high-risk mentally ill patients often migrate in a seemingly continuous manner between the mental health and the criminal justice system.

*Discharge Planning*

The forensic social worker in an assessment unit attends to discharge plans without really knowing what will occur in court. Organizing plans in advance presumes the judge will consider the individual eligible for bail or suitable for probation with an order to attend for treatment. The offender's motivation for help is another complicated issue. Since obtaining freedom from incarceration is usually a primary goal, many offenders initially agree to any and all referrals for rehabilitation and supportive housing because declaring an interest in help increases the likelihood of release. Unfortunately, once freedom is obtained, most offenders drop out of treatment and refuse all follow-up plans.

*Pretrial Assessments*

By consenting to or being ordered for a pretrial assessment, mentally ill offenders often spend more time confined for an offence than do non-mentally ill individuals. Understandably most mentally ill offenders resent the lengthy custodial arrangements, even if they understand why they have been charged. The new Criminal Code amendments (Bill C30), which specify length of time and reason for referral, and promote non-custodial assessments, are meant to address this problem. Also, the consequences of being found unfit for trial no longer imply indefinite custody; individuals found unfit will be admitted to psychiatric hospitals more rapidly for the treatment they require to proceed with their trials (Arnup & Siebenmorgen, 1992).

**Program Alternatives**

*Diversion*

A formalized diversion program, whereby the courts specifically request a report on the individual's needs and whether he or she is amenable to redirection to the mental health system, could legitimize what is already being done. It could sanction programs by investing the necessary time and funds to train staff who have an interest in coordinating treatment plans. A diversion program could occur after a brief out-patient assessment if the individual is willing to continue supervision, or after an in-patient stay once the person is stable enough to return to the community. This would require educating the patient about living skills and community resources, and linking him or her with follow-up. Specific contact people in the service network arranged for the patient could enable the family to follow the patient's progress, and the family could help the agencies coordinate plans for the patient.

A probation officer interested in working with mentally ill offenders could be seconded to consult on cases where an order for treatment is being considered as part of probation. Some boarding-houses could be designated for mentally ill offenders who are unable to decide where to live, until they go to court. Supervised boarding-homes are also needed in suburban communities and smaller cities, where many patients prefer to live.

One example of a diversion program model is the Hertfordshire Psychiatric Assessment Panel Scheme in rural England. The project, organized by a probation officer, has as fixed members a psychiatric nurse coordinator, a consultant psychiatrist and/or psychologist, and a probation officer. A social worker and other interagency staff become members as required. An individualized management plan that takes into consideration the person's illness and offending behaviour is implemented. If a crisis occurs, the panel can reconvene or return the individual to court for another sentence (Tonak, 1991).

*Case Management*

The Inter-Ministerial Project (IMP) is an assertive case-management program for chronic mentally ill individuals who have many problems, including conflicts with the law. This Vancouver program is staffed by five social workers, one of whom is the project coordinator, and a probation officer. The program is characterized by a long-term commitment to the client and frequent contacts with the client at home or on his or her own 'turf' (Wilson & Buckley, 1992). Office visits are avoided. The program has an evaluation component to assess whether the rate of rehospitalization or reincarceration is reduced and the quality of life increased. Although the research data collected to date are not sufficient to substantiate conclusions about the program's efficacy, the three-year follow-up phase should provide important information about the most useful services for this population.

It has long been argued that chronic psychiatric patients require as much individualized, comprehensive, continuous service in the community as they receive in hospital, and professionals need to be realistic in their expectations of these patients (Bachrach & Lamb, 1989: Wasylenki,

Plummer, & Littmann, 1981). Stein and Diamond (1985) have suggested that clinicians should help mentally ill patients accept responsibility for their recurring crimes by encouraging a brief period in jail as long as the family agrees and the mental health provider remains in contact with the patient and the prison staff.

## Summary

The relationship between the mental health and the criminal justice system is complicated. It has been affected by deinstitutionalization, changes in commitment laws and procedures, and the changing characteristics of patients admitted to hospitals. Decreased financial support for hospitals and increased attention to the community mental health movement have also had an effect. Further changes and challenges can be expected as a result of the recent Criminal Code amendments (Arnup & Siebenmorgen, 1992).

Teplin (1984) wrote that the criminal justice system was easily accessed and could not say 'no.' Other observers have noted that jail has become a mental hospital (Reeder & Meldman, 1991). Individuals 'rejected' by the mental health system readily 'accessed' the criminal justice system, but the difficulty was in returning them to the mental health stream after their release from custody (Johnson, 1990). Mentally ill offenders presented difficult operational issues, legal dilemmas, and philosophical paradoxes. Whether they were in jail or hospital, they were considered different and frequently were stigmatized (Jemelka, Trupin, & Chiles, 1989).

When the crimes committed are against the families of the mentally ill, social workers need to address the impact of the court proceedings on caregivers, review the options available through the court's authority, and simultaneously explore families' ambivalent, overwhelming feelings. This is a challenging task to accomplish in a brief, time-limited period, especially since psychosocial issues are not the primary mandate or concern of the court when a psychiatric assessment has been ordered.

Mentally ill offenders have a particularly difficult time, as do their chronic mentally ill counterparts, in the transition from an institution to the community (Bloom, Bradford, & Kofoed, 1988). The gains they make in an institutional setting are not readily transferable, especially when there is a gap between the systems and a lack of communication and coordination. Motivation to get help is questionable for many, and most housing and social agencies are reluctant to offer services to this group. Social workers need to be available to the family to answer questions that are posed about their relative and the court process itself. Assistance with navigating between the mental health and the criminal justice system provides needed support.

Pilot projects could be developed to reflect the multidisciplinary, multiservice approach. A diversion program, in which patients could be referred by the court for psychoeducational sessions on living skills, and families could participate to learn new coping strategies, may be effective for some pretrial forensic patients. These programs would need to include liaison and linkage with appropriate community services such as mental health clinicsand licensed boarding-homes. The solutions are not easy, but even small initiatives would ease the wait for an interministerial solution. Families need to be part of these plans because they are one of our most committed resources.

REFERENCES

Arnup, J., & Siebenmorgen, E. (1992 January). *Impact of Bill C-30 on METFORS*. Paper presented to Metfors. Toronto: Crown Law Office – Criminal.
Bachrach, L.L., & Lamb, R.H. (1989). Public psychiatry in an era of deinstitutionalization. In C.C. Beels & L.L. Bachrach (Eds.), *New directions for mental health services* (pp. 9–25). San Francisco: Jossey-Bass
Bloom, J.D., Bradford, J.M., & Kofoed, L. (1988). An overview of psychiatric treatment approaches to three offender groups. *Hospital and Community Psychiatry, 39*, 151–158.
Borzecki, M., & Wormith, J.S. (1985). The criminalization of psychiatrically ill people: A review with a Canadian perspective. *Psychiatric Journal of the University of Ottawa, 10* (4), 241–247.
Brennon, T.P., Gedrich, A.E., Jacoby, S.E., Tardy, M.J., & Tyson, K.B. (1986). Forensic social work: Practice and vision. *Social Casework: The Journal of Contemporary Social Work* (June), 340–350.
Cavanaugh, J.L., Wasyliw, O.E., & Rogers, R. (1990). Treatment of mentally disordered offenders. In G.L. Kleiman, M.M. Weissman, P.S. Appelbaum, & L.H. Roth. (Eds.), *Psychiatry: Vol. 3, Social, epidemiologic, and legal psychiatry*, 28 (Rev. ed.) (pp. 1–27). New York: Basic Books.
Hatfield, A.B. (1987a). Families as caregivers: A historical perspective. In A.B. Hatfield & H. Lefley (Eds.), *Families of the mentally ill: Coping and adaptation* (pp. 3–29). New York: Guilford.
Isaac, R.J., & Armat, V.C. (1990). *Madness in the street*. New York: Free Press.
Jemelka, R., Trupin, E., & Chiles, J.A. (1989). The mentally ill in prisons: A review. *Hospital and Community Psychiatry, 40*, 481–496.

Johnson, A.B. (1990). *Out of bedlam.* New York: Basic Books.

Lefley, H.P. (1987). The family's response to mental illness in a relative. In A.B. Hatfield (Ed), *New directions for mental health services* (pp. 3–21). San Francisco: Jossey-Bass.

McFarland, B.H., Faulkner, L.R., Bloom, J.D., Hallaux, R., & Bray, D.J. (1989). Chronic mental illness and the criminal justice system. *Hospital and Community Psychiatry, 40,* 718–723.

Reeder, D., & Meldman, L. (1991). Conceptualizing psychosocial nursing in the jail setting. *Journal of Psychosocial Nursing and Mental Health Services, 29* (8), 40–44.

Steadman, H.J., McCarty, D.W., & Morrissey, J.P. (1989). *The mentally ill in jail.* New York: Guilford.

Stein, L.I., & Diamond, R.J. (1985). The chronic mentally ill and the criminal justice system: When to call the police. *Hospital and Community Psychiatry, 36* (3), 271–274.

Teplin, L.A. (Ed.). (1984). *Mental health and criminal justice.* Beverly Hills: Sage Publications.

Tonak, D. (1991). *Psychiatric assessment panel scheme.* A paper presented at MET-FORS, Toronto.

Travis, S., & Protter, B. (1982). Mad or bad? Some clinical considerations in the misdiagnosis of schizophrenia as antisocial personality disorder. *American Journal of Psychiatry, 139,* 1335–1337.

Wasylenki, D.A., Plummer, E., & Littman, S. (1981). An aftercare program for problem patients. *Hospital and Community Psychiatry, 32,* 493–496.

Whitmer, G.E. (1980). From hospitals to jails: The fate of California's deinstitutionalized mentally ill. *American Journal of Orthopsychiatry, 50* (1), 65–75.

Wilson, D.A., & Buckley, R.L. (1992). Management of the multi-problem mentally disordered person: The inter-ministerial project: An assertive case management program. *British Columbia Medical Journal, 34* (4), 225–229.

# The Loss of a Child to Mental Illness

## APRIL COLLINS

Imagine what it would be like to have a member of your family afflicted with a condition whose sufferers, whenever the condition is depicted on TV, are portrayed as violent and homicidal. Imagine having your relatives obliquely avoid talking about the ill family member, unmistakably implying that your side of the family is guilty of something akin to Original Sin. (Johnson, 1988, p. xi)

The loss of a child to a schizophrenic illness is a painful reality for one in one hundred families (Sarason & Sarason, 1980). Fantasies that the bizarre, unpredictable behaviour is temporary must be abandoned and replaced with the reality that the illness, for most, will be controlled, not cured (Breier et al., 1991; Carone, Harrow, & Westermeyer, 1991). Schizophrenia, in spite of being the focus of research for decades, remains one of the most enigmatic and devastating of the psychiatric disorders (Kay, 1990). It is a disease that manifests itself during adolescence or early adulthood and is usually associated with a deterioration from a previous level of functioning (American Psychiatric Association, 1994). Attempts to establish an independent sense of self are often thwarted by disturbances of feeling and thought. Even if positive symptoms are controlled with psychotropic medication, social isolation, attentional impairment, an inability to feel intimate and amotivation persist for many, for decades (Cutting, 1986; Breier et al., 1991; Carone, Harrow, & Westermeyer, 1991).

Surprisingly few authors writing about schizophrenia have demonstrated an interest in issues related to the loss associated with mental illness; nor have they looked systematically at ways to help families mourn in a manner which encouraged healthy readjustment to their changed environment. Presumably, this lack is at least partially related to the tendency to look for the origins of schizophrenia within the family. In 1948, Fromm-Reichman first introduced the concept of the schizophrenogenic mother. The tradition of blaming the victims was later carried on by Bateson and colleagues (1956) with their double-bind hypothesis, and by Lidz, Fleck, and Cornelison (1965). These latter authors argued, for example, that schizophrenia occurred as a result of severe emotional strife within the family. Despite the lack of empirical evidence to support these etiological contentions, many professionals and lay people alike continue to adhere to these beliefs, and families continue to be viewed primarily as toxic. Recently, however, emphasis has shifted from the view of families as causal to the belief that they are agents who precipitate relapse (Lefley, 1989).

There is little doubt that, when a child is diagnosed with a chronic psychiatric illness like schizophrenia, there are painful and disorganizing consequences (Hatfield & Lefley, 1987). After the onset of the illness, life is invariably disturbed for disabled individuals and their families; the mentally ill family member likely faces a situation in which he or she will alternate for decades between acute psychotic states and periods of improvement or recovery (Wing, 1984). As well, families of the mentally ill often endure years of uncertainty, disappointment, guilt, and anguish.

There is general agreement that an extreme sense of loss can be expected among parents who learn that their child is disabled (Sargent & Liebman, 1985). This is based on the recognition that, for parents, the disability represents the loss of the wished-for normal child and of the known, previously non-disabled person (Hillyer-Davis, 1987; Solnit & Stark, 1961). A child is both a biological and a psychological extension of his or her parents (Rando, 1986). When an individual becomes mentally ill as an adolescent or young adult, parents have already accumulated an array of past images and experiences. This forms the basis on which they project future hopes for the child (Terkelsen, 1987). Once the chronic disabling condition strikes, the existing hopes, dreams, and expectations for the child, the family, and the future need to be mourned, while power, roles, and responsibilities are reassigned (Hatfield, 1987).

This essay argues, as did Miller and colleagues (1990), that grief is a significant, yet unrecognized dimension of the family's reaction to the changes in an ill relative. Unfortunately, the needs of families seem to be considered only to the extent necessary to stabilize the individual with schizophrenia (Titelman & Psyk, 1991). Furthermore, it is this author's contention that the plethora of information provided, in the spirit of 'psychoeducation,' does not, in any focused manner, address the ambivalence, guilt, and interminable sadness that overshadow issues for most families. This essay is a beginning attempt to fill the gap in the literature by examining the experience of and interventions for parents either struggling through or 'stuck' in an intense bereavement experience.

As with all losses, the meaning of the relationship to the mourner, the characteristics of that relationship, and the roles the child played determine what must be grieved by the bereaved parents (Rando, 1986). Many have described their experience as being 'like a death.' In fact, Miller and colleagues (1990), in a preliminary study, reported that families of the psychiatrically ill experience measurable grief, and that such grief may be comparable in magnitude to that suffered by those who have experienced a death. However, grief associated with chronic illness is perhaps in some ways more difficult. The lack of finality, for example, can hinder acceptance and allow the bereaved to cling to the hope that the disability will spontaneously remit. Additionally, not only does the disabled child not die, he also requires more care than do other children (Hillyer-Davis, 1987). Consequently, to 'resolve' grief in the traditional sense would require denial of the continuity of the child's life. Since the disabled child remains both physically and psychologically present, it is more helpful to consider family responses as natural reactions to an ongoing, often tragic experience – one that is not time-bound (Hillyer-Davis, 1987).

It seems reasonable to hypothesize that there are many reasons for parents to be exceptionally vulnerable to 'prolonged grief' when they lose a child to mental illness. Clinical experience demonstrates that most blame themselves for not protecting their child from the ravages of the illness. As well, they are generally inundated with a host of intense, unpleasant feelings. These can include but are not limited to: depression, anger, anxiety, guilt, and despair. Parental bereavement is also complicated by our socially prescribed expectations and responsibilities. There is a widespread belief that parents are to be all loving, totally selfless, and motivated only by the child and his or her welfare (Rando, 1986). These unattainable dictates can interfere with the normal expression of feelings of ambivalence, frustration, and anger that are a natural part of any relationship. Such feelings are not uncommon for parents of the mentally ill, but they are difficult to admit.

Mental illness in a child also strikes both partners in the marital dyad simultaneously. 'In a healthy relationship, each partner's most therapeutic resource is taken away, since the person to whom each would normally turn for support is deeply involved in his or her own grief. Not only must parents deal with the grief of their spouse but also their own sense of loss.

In light of the existing bond, there is little opportunity to get away from the grief, either psychologically or physically' (Rando, 1986, p. 25). One could further argue that the disruptions which are a natural part of any significant loss become potentially more damaging when spouses have pre-existing problems in their relationships. Ultimately the parents must master their grief concerning the child as well as those aspects of family life lost to the illness. The grieving process is continuous and may be reactivated at each developmental stage as the family becomes aware of the differences in the adult child and in the family life which are caused by the illness (Sargent & Liebman, 1985). However, it is important to distinguish between normal 'maturational grief' that may be triggered by life-cycle events and lingering unresolved grief – the product of an inadequate adaptation (Johnson & Rosenblatt, 1981).

No family style is inherently normal or abnormal (Minuchin, 1974). Rather, style is influenced by the family's own history, composition, developmental stage, and subculture. Of importance is the adaptive value of the responses families use when challenged with the threat of schizophrenia. Some are remarkably resourceful – they are able to work out new patterns of living and emerge from the grief imposed by their losses in a healthy manner (Worden, 1982). In these instances, families have not achieved a total triumph over the schizophrenic illness, nor have they surrendered to it, but, rather, they have reached a compromise which, to them, is acceptable (White, 1985). At the same time, others fail to demonstrate this impressive resilience. These families do not meet the new demands with creative solutions, nor have they adapted old strategies to meet the challenges of the current situation (ibid.). Instead, they get 'stuck,' using habitual patterns of interaction, as they attempt to re-establish equilibrium within their boundaries following the onset of the illness. 'These families remain interminably in a state of grief without progression of the mourning ... they DO NOT move toward assimilation or accommodation but, instead, are locked into stereotyped repetitions which interrupt healing' (Horowitz et al., 1980, p. 1157).

Clinical observations have suggested that 'triangulated' families (Haley, 1976) are particularly vulnerable to long-term disruption and dysfunction when faced with the threat of schizophrenia. They are often paralysed by their grief – unable to move beyond it. It is noteworthy that triangles do not exist only in the families of people with schizophrenia. Nor are they the product of psychiatric illness. Rather, it appears that these transactional preferences exist in families prior to the onset of illness. These dynamics may be present covertly and in a way that does not grossly impair everyday functioning within the family. However, with the onset of a severe schizophrenic illness, familiar and preferred ways of responding seem to work to inhibit successful resolution of grief and subsequent adaptation. This author speculates that this particular dynamic does not permit members to move through the tasks of mourning that are necessary. The system as a whole is strongly invested in restoring relationships that existed premorbidly.

Triangulated families tend to be enmeshed and display closed and rigid external boundaries. They isolate themselves from outside sources and influences. At the same time, internal subsystem boundaries are diffuse and poorly defined, and there is no clear parental alliance. In these instances, the parental relationship tends to be empty, and the child inadvertently fills the needs that would ordinarily have been satisfied by the marital partner in a healthier marriage. A coalition between one spouse and the child is reinforced, and a feed-back loop is established (Dawson, Munroe-Blum, & Bartolucci, 1983). The child and the parent reciprocally influence each other in an ongoing pattern of mutual reinforcement.

Unfortunately, in many instances, this same group of families appears to become victimized over time by the child with schizophrenia. As the illness evolves, the pre-existing, disturbed power relationships within the family become increasingly distorted. The afflicted child acts out his own grief and frustration in the only way he knows how – by behaving in a regressed, abusive manner. He, too, is invested in restoring the relationships that existed prior to the onset of the illness, the one that had been secure and predictable, the one in which he had been in charge.

**Treatment Approach**

In formulating the treatment approach for triangulated families with a tyrannical member afflicted with schizophrenia, this author's work has been strongly influenced by the structural (Minuchin, 1974), focal family (Levene, Jeffries, & Newman, 1984), and grief (Worden, 1982; Rando, 1986) theories. Here, there are at least two broad goals. First, and foremost, abusive behaviour must be modified and independence in the regressed child must be encouraged. Attempts are then made to facilitate the process of normal grieving in families where a loss to schizophrenia has occurred. Ideally, family members are able to negotiate a balance between proceeding with their lives and recognizing and accepting the demands imposed by the chronic illness (Sargent & Liebman, 1985).

In keeping with Minuchin's (1987) work, optimally parents need to function as the executive subsystem that makes decisions for the family. They must work together to make parenting decisions about the behaviour that will and will not be tolerated in their interactions with their children. Clearly, in triangulated families this does not occur. Rather, subsystem boundaries around the spouses are diffuse, and consequently are subject to intrusion by children. As long as these boundaries remain unclear, the abusive behaviour remains permissible. To achieve the first goal, clinicians must redraw the boundaries within the family. The parental subsystem needs to be strengthened so spouses can negotiate spouse issues without involving the child with schizophrenia. At the same time, the boundary that protects the child and encourages autonomy must be clearly defined. Under these circumstances, the person with schizophrenia needs help to individuate. If the child is left in the triangle, a satisfactory ego identity fails to develop and he or she remains in an enmeshed, dysfunctional coalition.

Parents in such families typically present to clinicians as frustrated, angry, and exhausted. Often their chief complaint is that their child is 'out of control' and they want the clinician to 'fix' the problem. A concrete behavioural approach has proven to be most useful as a first-line defence against acting-out behaviour. To increase the probability of success, a thorough understanding of the problem behaviour is required. This includes details concerning the conditions under which acting-out is likely to occur, the function of the behaviour within the family, and the personal characteristics of the abusive individual that might contribute to the problem behaviour (i.e., the person does not have alternative interpersonal skills). When the clinician has this information, a statement of the specific changes that are desired can be negotiated and operationalized. Consequences for acting-out or failure to comply are established. The clinician is directive, and, with the afflicted individual present, the parents are empowered and encouraged to 'take charge.' As in focal family therapy, it is suggested that parents make decisions for their child until he or she is able to assume this responsibility. Ideally the situation stabilizes over time, and the child with schizophrenia goes on to function in a more self-directed way.

It is at this point that clinical work shifts from family to individual and couples therapy. The focus of treatment turns to mourning the losses associated with the schizophrenic illness. Without this component of treatment, there is an increased likelihood that the child with schizophrenia and the parents will remain bound in an emotionally unhealthy manner. Using a variation of grief theory, sessions proceed by: (1) helping the child and parents accept the reality of the illness and its implications;

(2) facilitating the expression of affect; and (3) identifying and working-through impediments to readjustment.

Clinically, achieving the third goal is often the most arduous task. Both the parents and the child are invested in trying to get back the relationships that existed premorbidly. Consequently, getting stuck in terms of accepting the reality of the illness is not uncommon. While they openly speak of schizophrenia, they are unable to entertain the possibility that the illness is chronic and will not go away. Instead, they search longingly for the cure. After all, a cure would allow the family to return to more familiar and comfortable relationships.

What follows is a case example of one of the families the author worked with in clinical practice.

*Case History*

Barbara, a twenty-seven-year-old single female was admitted to an in-patient psychiatric ward for approximately 6.5 months in 1989, following a physical assault against her mother. She had no insight, remained amotivational, and regularly blamed her parents for her illness. Barbara had been diagnosed with schizophrenia in 1984, at age twenty-two, and had had ten admissions since that time. Her behaviour at home had become more aggressive, with outbursts increasing in frequency and intensity. Verbal threats and physically assaultive behaviour were common during interactions with her parents, though most of the violence was directed towards her mother. Inadequacy, sadness, inferiority, and hopelessness were prominent and recurrent themes for Barbara. She was fully cognizant of the disabilities that had been imposed by her illness. Barbara was an only child. Her early years and adolescence were said to be unremarkable, though she was described as a stubborn child who would not listen. Her parents had been married for approximately thirty years. Mr T., the breadwinner, worked long hours and was involved in many activities outside the home in his spare time. He had an autocratic personal style and was rigid, non-supportive, controlled, and very controlling. He was described as being critical by both his wife and his daughter. There was no clear parental alliance in the marriage. Mrs T. was the homemaker and was responsible for childrearing. Mrs T. and Barbara were allies from an early age. Mrs T. served as a buffer for Barbara when Mr T. was imposing decisions. Barbara, in turn, was used by her mother as an emotional substitute for her husband. The coalition between the two was best described as reciprocally dependent. Mrs T. was excessively invested in her parenting role because there was little else in her life. Barbara had always had few limits set for her and had not been encouraged to assume responsibility within the family. She had not been allowed to experiment with growing up, and was an indulged child.

Following the onset of her illness, Barbara's behaviour at home worsened progressively until it reached tyrannical proportions. When asked to do something, she would respond by throwing a temper tantrum. She would often threaten to kill her parents or to set the house on fire. Sometimes she would break household items and/or attack her parents. Mr and Mrs T. would react in a predictable manner. Her father would stand and scream back at her. At the height of anger he had once told Barbara that she had ruined his life. In turn, Mr T. would accuse his wife of being weak and unable to throw Barbara out of the house permanently. Typically, following such an attack, Mr T. would leave the premises for several hours at a time. Mrs T., on the other hand, would apologize to Barbara for making whatever demand had led to the outburst. She would reach out and try to comfort Barbara and denounce her husband's behaviour. Neither parent had any insight into the way that his or her behaviour was contributing to Barbara's aggressiveness. They frequently blamed the hospital staff, claiming that the prescribed medication was responsible for the behaviour problems.

As suggested earlier, the goals with these kinds of families are twofold. First and foremost, abusive behaviour needs to be reduced (or, ideally, eliminated) while, simultaneously, independence is facilitated in the regressed adult child. Additionally, since triangulated families tend to behave in ways which seem to inhibit successful adaptation to loss, therapy also needs to be directed towards facilitating the tasks of mourning. In this case example, the first goal was achieved through the use of a concrete behavioural approach. Practically this meant that Barbara's parents were educated about her illness and prognosis. They were then encouraged to look at the way their mixed messages were contributing to and perpetuating the problem. The need to work together was identified and strongly emphasized to the couple.

In keeping with the philosophy of focal family therapy (Levene, Newman, & Jeffries, 1989), the problems were reframed for the family. They were encouraged to view limit-setting, not as punitive, but as a way of demonstrating concern, and to recognize that Barbara needed to learn more appropriate ways to express her feelings. The were also encouraged to let Barbara grow up and assume responsibility for herself and her actions.

The parents were then assisted in establishing a set of rules and expectations for their daughter when she was home on weekend passes. The family were cautioned to expect Barbara to act-out initially. Again, it was useful to normalize this by explaining that it is not uncommon to see testing behaviour when limits are set. Once the parents were in agreement about their expectations, Barbara was invited into the sessions with her parents and was asked to provide input regarding what she thought was reasonable in terms of the proposed rules and expectations. Barbara agreed and understood that weekend passes to her parents' home would be contingent upon compliance with negotiated rules. The period that followed was a particularly stressful time for the couple because they were asserting themselves in a way they never had before. As predicted, Barbara did act-out aggressively. Her parents had difficulty working together and, at times, reverted to their previous ways of relating to each other and Barbara, and Mrs T. suffered the most with self-imposed guilt. She was conflicted around the issue of setting limits versus giving her 'poor sick child' anything she wanted. Whenever Mrs T. was unable to follow through with the limits she had established, she would insist that she had to give in, as her priority was to give her daughter a few minutes of pleasure. Falling back to the old way of doing things was safe and easy and kept her from being overwhelmed by guilt.

Obviously, this process is never a smooth one; invariably there are failures because one part of the system breaks down. It is most important to support the family by addressing their concerns and fears and renegotiating strategies for change when necessary. With time and consistent application, this approach can be useful and beneficial to families.

Only after a long, hard struggle did Barbara's behaviour lose some of its power within the context of her family. Once she began to emancipate herself from her parents, Barbara was offered and welcomed individual sessions. Initially work focused on helping her to examine her own feelings about her illness. There was little doubt that Barbara was suffering. She, too, had to grieve the loss of her hopes, dreams, and expectations of herself. Barbara was truly ambivalent. She was afraid to be ill and afraid to be well. Being well necessitated 'growing up,' a process that happens neither quickly nor easily. Eventually she was better able to accept her illness and her limitations but continued to have difficulty establishing more realistic goals for herself. At the time Barbara was referred for individual psychotherapy, her parents were offered couples work around the same issue. Mrs T. expressed an interest in this, but her husband refused. He was 'too busy to take time off.' Mrs T. had previously noted that, during every one of Barbara's hospitalizations, the marriage had been identified as problematic.

Interestingly Mrs T. had made it perfectly clear from the outset that, while she realized that the marriage had problems, she was not prepared to do anything about it. What she did agree to do was meet with the writer individually and talk about Barbara, who she was and what she had been like before she got sick. She spoke in great detail about the things that they used to enjoy doing together and recalled some of her fondest memories. Once the foundation of positive memories was established, Mrs T. was able to begin to look at some of the ambivalent feelings and memories. She expressed anxiety and a strong desire to have things return to the way they used to be. She was able to link this with her own fear that she would be left alone, with nothing to replace her relationship with Barbara. Her feelings of guilt were discussed in great detail. Therapy also focused on all that she had given Barbara prior to the onset of her illness and all that she could continue to give her. Mrs T. needed to mourn the loss of the future that she had hoped for herself and Barbara. Perhaps her most difficult challenge was to pull back emotionally and reinvest some energy in other relationships. In many ways, these tasks seem to be mutually incompatible – she was being asked to simultaneously hold on to and let go of the relationship she had with her daughter.

## Summary

When a child is diagnosed with a chronic psychiatric illness like schizophrenia, parents can and do experience an extreme sense of loss. Unfortunately, their grief has not been adequately recognized or addressed by clinicians. Families have not been afforded the opportunity to mourn their existing hopes, dreams, and expectations for their child. Instead, their dilemmas have been considered only to the extent necessary to meet the needs of the 'system.'

This essay attempts to argue that grief is a significant issue that needs to be discussed. Social workers are in a particularly good position to offer this kind of service to families. Ultimately the goal should be to help families learn to live with the tragedy of mental illness to the best of their ability. This cannot be achieved unless 'mourning' is addressed in a thoughtful and sensitive manner.

REFERENCES

American Psychiatric Association. 1994. *Diagnostic and Statistical Manual of Mental Disorders, Fourth Edition, Revised.* Washington, DC: Author.

Bateson, G., Jackson, D., Haley, J., & Weakland, J. (1956). Toward a theory of schizophrenia. *Behavioural Science, 1*, 251–264.

Breier, A., Schreiber, J., Dyer, J., & Pickar, D. (1991). National Institute of Mental Health longitudinal study of chronic schizophrenia. *Archives of General Psychiatry, 48*, 239–246.

Carone, B., Harrow, M., & Westermeyer, J. (1991). Posthospital course and outcome in schizophrenia. *Archives of General Psychiatry, 48*, 247–253.

Cutting, J. (1986). *The psychology of schizophrenia.* New York: Churchill Livingstone.

Dawson, D., Munroe-Blum, H., & Bartolucci, G. (1983). *Schizophrenia in focus.* New York: Human Services Press.

Fromm-Reichman, F. (1948). Notes on the development of treatment of schizophrenia by psychoanalytic psychotherapy. *Psychiatry, 11*, 263–273.

Hatfield, A., & Lefley, H. (1987). *Families of the mentally ill: Coping and adaptation.* New York: Guilford.

Haley, J. (1976). *Problem-solving therapy: New strategies for effective family therapy* (1st ed.). San Francisco: Jossey-Bass

Hillyer-Davis, B. (1987). Disability and grief. *Social Casework: The Journal of Contemporary Social Work, 68*, 352–357.

Horowitz, M., Wilner, M., Marmar, C., & Krupnick, J. (1980). Pathological grief and the activation of latent self-images. *The American Journal of Psychiatry, 137*, 1157–1162.

Johnson, J. (1988). *Hidden victims: An eight stage healing process for families and friends of the mentally ill.* Toronto: Doubleday.

Johnson, P., & Rosenblatt, P. (1981). Grief following childhood loss of a parent. *American Journal of Psychotherapy, 35*, 419–425.

Kay, S. (1990). Significance of the positive–negative distinction in schizophrenia. *Schizophrenia Bulletin, 16*, 635–652.

Lefley, H. (1989). Family burden and family stigma in major mental illness. *American Psychologist, 44*, 556–560.

Levene, J., Jeffries, J.J., Newman, F. (1984). Focal family therapy: A component in the treatment of schizophrenia. *International Journal of Family Psychiatry, 5* (1), 3–19.

Levene, J., Newman, F., & Jeffries, J. J. (1989). Focal family outcome study I: Patient and family functioning. *Canadian Journal of Psychiatry, 34*, 641–647.

Lidz, T., Fleck, S., & Cornelison, A. (1965). *Schizophrenia and the family.* New York: International Universities Press.

Miller, F., Dworkin, J., Ward, M., & Barone, D. (1990). A preliminary study of unresolved grief in families of seriously mentally ill patients. *Hospital & Community Psychiatry, 41*, 1321–1325.

Minuchin, S. (1974). *Families and family therapy*. Cambridge, MA: Harvard University Press.

Rando, T. (1986). *Parental loss of a child*. Champagne, IL: Research Press Company.

Sarason, I., & Sarason, B. (1980). *Abnormal psychology*. Englewood Cliffs, NJ: Prentice-Hall.

Sargent, J., & Liebman, R. (1985). Childhood chronic illness: Issues for psychotherapists. *Community Mental Health Journal, 21* (1), 294–311.

Solnit, A., & Stark, M. (1961). Mourning and the birth of a defective child. *Psychoanalytic Study of the Child, 16,* 523–537.

Terkelsen, K. (1987). The evolution of family responses to mental illness through time. In A. Hatfield & H. Lefley (Eds.), *Families of the mentally ill: Coping and adaptation* (pp. 151–166). New York: Guilford.

Titelman, D., & Psyk, L. (1991) Grief, guilt and identification in siblings of schizophrenic individuals. *Bulletin of the Menninger Clinic, 55,* 72–84.

White, R. (1985). Strategies of adaptation: An attempt at systematic description. In A. Monat & R. Lazarus (Eds.), *Stress and coping* (pp. 121–144). New York: Columbia University Press.

Wing, J.K. (1984). Long-term social adaptation in schizophrenia. In N. Miller & G. Cohen (Eds.), *Schizophrenia & aging* (pp. 183–205). New York: Guilford.

Worden, W. (1982). *Grief counselling and grief therapy*. New York: Springer.

# The Forgotten Sibling

## DAVE DENBERG

Time stands still. This could be last year, or the year before or the year before that. I'm within range of becoming a physician, while my brother still dreams of having a small job, living in his own apartment and of being well. I recall an evening some time ago when I drove (home) to tell my parents and my brother that I was getting married. My brother's eyes lit up at the news, and then a darkness fell over them.

'What's wrong?' I asked him.

'It's funny,' he answered matter-of-factly. 'You're getting married and I've never even had a girlfriend.' My mother's eyes filled with tears, and she turned away. She was trying her best to be happy for me, for the dreams I had, for the dreams so many of us take for granted.

'You still have us,' I stammered touching his arm.

All of a sudden my dreams meant nothing; I didn't deserve them and they weren't worth talking about. My brother shrugged his shoulders, smiled and shook my hand, his large tobacco-stained fingers wrapping around my hand, dwarfing it. (Aronowitz, 1988)

Sibling relationships have received little attention in the study and treatment of serious psychiatric disorders. With few exceptions, most clinical literature refers either globally to 'the family' or specifically to 'parents.' A handful of authors differentiate the experience and needs of well siblings, and fewer still (often themselves siblings of a mentally ill brother or sister) have written about the sibling experience.

Why has this topic received so little attention in the literature? There are many possible explanations. Clearly contributory is the relative invisibility of siblings and the infrequency of their involvement in the consultation process or in family conferences. Often an implicit assumption by professionals is that successfully engaging and helping parents provides the family as a whole with the resources it needs to cope with illness or crisis situations. Parents also often describe well siblings as being disengaged from the person with the illness. They seem to want to protect 'well' siblings from further disruption to their lives and often feel that the problem is their responsibility. Finally, the complexity of sibling relationships has not been fully explored, let alone understood. Thus, there is no context which establishes the onset and recurrence of a chronic mental illness as a significant event in a sibling's life. In many ways siblings of the mentally ill have been 'forgotten.'

## The Sibling Relationship

Historically the sibling relationship has received some attention in theoretical, empirical, and observational studies. However, several characteristics of this literature have limited its usefulness in offering a comprehensive understanding of sibling relationships and their significance. First and foremost, many authors have tended to focus on a particular topic of interest (such as birth order, sibling rivalry, twin studies) and have examined it from their particular perspective (i.e., psychoanalysis, family-systems theory, sociology, or developmental psychology). There has been no unifying theory that could integrate these discrete perspectives (Bank & Kahn, 1982). They have also tended to focus on a particular phase of development (e.g., childhood) and have examined either the immediate impact or the later developmental significance of events that occurred earlier in life. Unfortunately, a comprehensive understanding of the nature of the sibling relationship, with both its enduring effects and an ongoing dynamic developmental process, has been absent. Bank and Kahn (1982) made a beginning attempt to integrate the literature, and have offered a significant, although necessarily incomplete, contribution to understanding this topic.

### The Contribution of Bank and Kahn: The Sibling Bond

Bank and Kahn (1982) combined an exhaustive review of the literature available in 1982 with the results of their own intensive interviews with sibling groups and their observation of sibling themes which had emerged in individual psychotherapy. They sought to synthesize the available knowledge and make some beginning attempts to work towards the development of a comprehensive theory of the sibling relationship. They also began to clarify its place in relation to parental influence.

These authors postulated that a 'sibling bond' exists and that it receives its initial impetus and intensity from the degree of 'access' which siblings have to one another (Bank & Kahn, 1982). They argued that siblings raised together, who are close in age, spend a lot of time together over a period of years, share friends, and have more intense bonds. Furthermore, they postulated that this bond went beyond social and peripheral aspects of personality to the core self. The sibling bond is a stable, continuous essence which cannot be verbalized or consciously understood (Bank & Kahn, 1982). The bond can be positive, negative, or mixed, based on the degree of congruence between the identity needs of the siblings. In early childhood, it is greatly influenced by factors largely outside of the children's control, including, but not limited to, parental fantasies or wishes about the relationship between the children, and the way the parents behave towards them as 'the kids,' 'the boys,' 'the girls,' and as individuals. This bond is also said to influence such processes as identity formation with respect to the sexual and aggressive drives (Bank & Kahn, 1982). Sibling aggression and rivalry may be a positive source of vitality, self-definition, and motivation for learning interpersonal skills, or may take crippling and damaging forms. Sexual identity may be highly affected by identification, rivalry, or disgust with a sibling, leading to emulation, differentiation, or the choice of an alternate identity (e.g., 'The Brain' when another sister is already 'The Beauty'). Siblings may remain a basis of comparison for each other in adulthood, affecting each other's sense of personal worth in areas such as achievement and success, sexuality and beauty, and social and family relationships (Bank & Kahn, 1982).

One premise underlying this discussion is that there is reliable, consistent parental care or a suitable replacement adult figure. This allows the primary consolidation of aspects of identity to occur in relation to the parents. When parents die, abandon their children, or are emotionally unavailable or disturbed in their parenting function, and there is no one to take their place, a pathological variant of the 'sibling bond' occurs (Bank & Kahn, 1982). The bonds intensify, whether in a positive or negative direction, and may take on excessive importance. The result may be an intensely close, mutually supportive, and reciprocally loyal sibling group whose members derive identity, pleasure, comfort, and support. This extreme variant comes at the cost of exclusion of others and constriction of choices available to the members of the sibling group. Alternatively, one sibling may assume the role of caretaker, perhaps at the cost of rigidity, inhibition of growth, and personality constriction for all siblings in the family. Other extreme patterns include incest, violence within the sibling group, intense competition, fragmentation of the group, or a frozen, polarized image of a sibling which is subsequently very difficult to alter.

Bank and Kahn consider the normal sibling bond in adulthood as one in which there is partial identification with a sense of the self and sibling as separate persons, similar in some ways and different in others. The relationship may contain a dialectical balance between positive and negative feelings. Most important, the bond is not excessively intense or central to the point of personality constriction. Pathological bonds are characterized by excessive closeness in which the sense of self is blurred or lost, or by excessive distance resulting in rejection or disowning of the sibling (Bank & Kahn, 1982).

## Siblings from Other Perspectives

### The Literature on Child Development

Some interesting new results are emerging in the area of child development. Here, careful empirical study has suggested that the area is more complex than had previously been thought. Some investigators have argued, for example, that a distinction can be made between studies done by clinicians (including Bank & Kahn, 1982) and empirical researchers (Dunn & Plomin, 1991). It has been suggested that the former take samples from the population of 'disturbed' families, whereas the latter have examined sibling processes in 'normal' families. They have cautioned that the discontinuity between these populations may not be fully known, and the study of an individual sibling (whether empirically or in psychotherapy) may yield a different result from the study of that same person in the context of his or her sibling group. Moreover, much of the data that are presented in the literature are correlational without proving cause, influenced by mediating variables, and at times can be interpreted in the light of contradictory theories (Dunn, 1992).

### The Literature on Adult Development

Recent work in the field of adult development supports Bank and Kahn's (1982) belief that the basic nature of the sibling bond is established early in life but can be influenced by the current relationship between adult siblings (Gold, 1989). One study reported, for example, that 'critical incidents' during the lifetime can have a differential impact on siblings, depending upon the previous quality of the relationship (Ross & Milgram, 1982). Specifically, major negative incidents did not ultimately damage good relationships; however, seemingly minor problems could potentially maintain or increase conflict in already troubled ones. Ross and Milgram (1982) also noted that closeness, conflict, rivalry, and other sibling processes are affected by the ongoing influence of the parents, the emotional climate and value system within the family, each sibling's adherence to or rejection of it, and normative developmental change.

According to Goetting (1986), the developmental tasks for siblings vary across the life cycle, with some remaining constant (such as companionship, emotional support, and the provision of aid and direct services), while others vary with the stage of the life cycle (such as delegated caretaking in childhood and adolescence, and the care of an elderly parent). Further support for this contention comes from a retrospective study of sibling relationships across the life span. Gold (1989) found that these relationships possess features of both continuity and dynamic flexibility into the final decade of the life span.

## Siblings in the Psychoanalytic Literature

Until recently, the psychoanalytic literature on sibling relationships focused primarily on envy, rivalry, and jealousy (Colonna & Newman, 1983). While sibling influences in these areas were seen as affecting aspects of identity formation, character development, and object choice, they were seen as secondary in importance to, and determined by the experience with, parents. However, intensive observational studies of very young children with siblings a few years older have demonstrated that older siblings exert significant influence on the younger's negotiation of the separation–individuation process, and that this is, to a degree, independent of the parental influence (Neubauer, 1983). Other authors identify sibling contributions to early development both with respect to the management of aggressive and sexual drives and in areas of autonomous ego functioning (Kris & Ritvo, 1983). In relation to Oedipal conflict, the older sibling acts as an alternative to the attraction to Mother, thus potentially both easing the intensity of the process while perhaps making it more complicated (ibid.). These authors all identify a significant component of empathic identification between siblings as a normal and important part of separation–individuation (Leitchman, 1985; Provence &

Solnit, 1983). Thus, while reaffirming the primacy of the parental influence and identifying various other factors, these studies argue that the sibling influence on personality development is significant. That siblings have a profound and lasting influence is further evidenced by the revival of sibling themes in a mother expecting a second child (Abarbanel, 1983), and in both parents' expectations and treatment of their own children (Kris & Ritvo, 1982; Jacobson, cited in Colonna & Newman, 1983). Neubauer (1983) suggests that careful attention should be paid, not only to the phase-specific influence of the sibling relationships, but also to the way it changes over the course of the life cycle.

Graham (1988) reviewed sibling-related material from thirty-five cases in his adult analytic practice. He commented on the need during these analyses to maintain separate images of the sibling relationship as an inner complex of roles and relationships and as a current, real relationship in the patient's life. He suggested that siblings have considerable significance, not only phenomenologically, but also in the development of psychic structure. Powerful effects occurred in relation to sibling attachment; sibling rivalry; lost, damaged, or frustrating siblings; and loving and incestuous ties. Siblings who took restorative or mediating roles in the family tended to internalize these as an enduring part of their personality. Graham also argued that siblings need to separate and individuate from each other as well as from parents. He concluded that there is a separate line of development which, from earliest childhood, operates along with infantile attachments to and separations from both parents. The ideal end-point of this process is when siblings are able to reaffirm their bonds with affectionate celebration of each other's achievement of independence, equality, and connection.

In summary, sibling relationships are neither simple nor unimportant. The significance that a given sibling holds in a person's life is the product of an intricate process of development within the context of family. No comprehensive theory exists at this time to integrate all the available information. However, the actual current relationship between adult siblings seems anchored in a natural ebb and flow related to life-cycle tasks, and is coloured by family factors and variables specific to the relationship between the siblings. All authors, regardless of their conceptual framework, seem to agree that parents are and should be the primary figures in a child's development, and that their displacement by sibling bonds is a pathological variant. However, for at least some, siblings retain unconscious significance, and this serves as an organizer of certain kinds of major life experience (Graham, 1988; Kris & Ritvo, 1982; Abarbanel,

1983; Colonna & Newman, 1983). Both the actual current adult relationship between the siblings and the unconscious dimension are important, and it can be difficult to separate the two (Graham, 1988).

Any given sibling relationship, whether close and supportive, rivalrous and conflicted, or apparently peripheral and innocuous, is a product of these important and complex processes. Psychiatric illness in a sibling intrudes on this relationship.

### Siblings of the Mentally Ill

While the literature on siblings of the mentally ill is not well developed, several significant shifts in thinking about this relationship have occurred over the years. The work of early investigators (Lidz et al., 1963; Newman, 1966; Meissner, 1970) was strongly influenced by the prevailing belief that schizophrenia was caused by pathological family processes. Clearly, they reasoned, if family pathology was the major causative factor, all siblings should become ill. However, it became obvious very quickly that not all siblings were affected, and consequently these researchers were forced to explain this paradox. Some argued that siblings were significantly disturbed, just not schizophrenic (Lidz et al., 1963; Samuels & Chase, 1979), while others offered theoretical explanations which identified specific processes that would predict which sibling became ill (Newman, 1966). In direct contrast, others presented results which suggested that siblings of those afflicted with schizophrenia were no different from young persons in the general population (Hoover & Franz, 1972).

In the past ten to fifteen years, it has been established that family processes do not cause schizophrenia (Waring et al., 1986). Consequently, there has been a shift in the literature on families of patients with schizophrenia. Instead of attempting to uncover the roots of family pathology, the current literature examines the experience of having and caring for a mentally ill family member, the burdens posed by this situation, and the needs of families as they struggle to manage. More recently, a number of authors have looked specifically at the impact of mental illness on siblings (Landeen et al., 1992; Riebschleger, 1991; Titleman & Psyk, 1991). A number of common themes have emerged. Specifically, these studies have suggested that clinicians be aware of, and attend to, the emotional and intrapsychic needs of persons when they are coming to terms with schizophrenia in a sibling (Titleman & Psyk, 1991; Riebschleger, 1991; Johnson, 1988). The needs of siblings as caretakers or members of the ill person's support network (Landeen et al., 1992; Riebschleger, 1991) and the need to balance the sibling's own life with involvement in the patient's and family's struggle must also be addressed (Bank & Kahn, 1982; Johnson, 1988). The first-person and anecdotal accounts presented below also vividly highlight a fourth theme, that of 'invisible baggage,' the emotional and psychological burden of having an ill sibling

Recently some attention has been given to those factors which affect the ease with which a well sibling manages the direct 'caretaker' role. The age and developmental stage of the well sibling when the disturbing behaviour first occurs, the rate of onset and chronicity of the disturbed sibling's problems, and the degree of embarrassment or stigma resulting from the disturbed sibling's behaviour have been implicated as significant factors which influence adjustment (Bank & Kahn, 1982). Riebschleger (1991) also argued that stress in a sibling's own personal life, difficulty accepting the loss of a brother or sister, the cyclical nature of the illness, mixed messages from the mental health system around responsibility, and being included in the patient's delusional system tended to exacerbate difficulties with the caregiving role. Siblings reported suffering particularly from mixed emotions, in which anger at the ill sibling and the family conflicted with survivor guilt. Riebschleger's respondents had considerable direct involvement in the support and instrumental assistance of their ill sibling, and many felt that the mental health system had not adequately addressed the pain and trauma they had experienced. The studies by Riebschleger (1991) and Landeen and colleagues (1992) are unusual in that they asked siblings directly about their needs. In 1992, Landeen and her colleagues conducted a needs assessment and found that respondents expressed the desire for information about the illness and its long-term management, and requested programs which would help facilitate communication between family members and the ill relative. Siblings expressed concern for the future and wondered about the degree of independence, satisfaction, and quality of life that was possible for their ill brother or sister. Of note is that those respondents whose relatives were in treatment reported little intrusion of the illness into their own lives. This is in direct contrast to those siblings whose relatives were tenuously or completely uninvolved in treatment. It appears that the stability of the patient from the standpoint of the illness significantly influences the perception of needs.

The following self-reports vividly convey various aspects of the sibling experience of psychiatric illness:

When I moved to Colorado I was able to forget their daily struggle and pursue my own. But every now and then I'd hear he was in some hospital, either the best

(Cornell's New York Hospital in White Plains) or Creedmore State. It didn't matter all that much in the long run; each was a nightmare for him, and neither cured him or provided prolonged relief ... He'd always try and sometime manage a smile through his blackened, deepset eyes when I'd visit him from Colorado in his final years. But he had given up most ties to people from the normal world, and he spent his time within his mind and with those who shared his brand of isolation. I'd sit with him for a while; neither he nor I could bear to sit together for long. I'd take off his glasses and clean them while he told me of his latest desperate realizations, and I'd wonder where the little boy I'd loved so dearly had gone. (Jaffe, 1992)

Every Sunday night my family has a dinner where we exchange stories and share what our plans are for the coming week. Mark used to tell such grand stories of what he was learning in college and whom he met. But since he got sick and spent a summer in the hospital, he sits quietly at the end of the table, his eyes focused on his plate, sometimes mumbling to himself. I once asked him to tell a story, but he got angry and left the table. No one talks about his summer in the hospital. No one asks him what his day was like or if he had plans for the week. But I keep going to our Sunday dinners hoping Mark will tell us another one of his stories, hoping this time Mark will look up at me and smile. (Johnson, 1988)

It is now about a decade since Andy was first diagnosed as schizophrenic. I no longer feel that my brother and I are shadow-sides of the same person or that our destinies are entwined. On the deepest level where intellect leaves off and great emotion begins, I know I am not Andy. Today, I can see him without fear, but not without sorrow. The chronic nature of his illness makes it a problem that is never truly resolved, and the sadness I feel about the bleakness of his life is a burden I still carry around like invisible luggage ...

When I remember the closeness Andy and I shared as children, the memory often seems dim, almost illusionary, as though it not only happened in another time, but in another realm, to two other people. (Brodoff, 1988)

When, a few years later, she knocked a mirror over onto my pet lizard, cutting off his tail, I was horrified. When I think about that night I view the scene as if I were watching a film; the crying child I was looks like an unfamiliar actress. Although I never withdrew to the extent that those suffering from multiple personality disorder do, I had learned the trick of backing away within my body to hide in some small corner of the self.

... Part of the healing, I have come to accept, is recognizing how good my instincts were. Hiding, pacifying, coddling my siblings when I could – these and other traits we all learned in those madhouses do not suit us now, but they may have saved our lives then. Perhaps, I think R.D. Laing was right in theory but named the wrong sibling. As the sisters and brothers of schizophrenics, we may exhibit bizarre behaviour, but we are sane. We're the ones who developed healthy responses to an unhealthy world. (Simon, 1993)

*Emotional and Intrapsychic Processes*

Most authors generally agree that siblings struggle with feelings such as fear of becoming ill, survivor guilt, the sense of stigma, and anger and shame (Bank & Kahn, 1982; Newman, 1966; Harris, 1988). Many believe that they have caused the illness or are not doing enough to help. They mourn the loss of their normal family and what might have been. Siblings face a painful dilemma, one in which they have to draw the line when their own needs compete with those of the patient and family. Riebschleger (1991) suggested that there are parallels between what siblings of the mentally ill experience and what Kübler-Ross (1969) described when a person is forced to come to terms with death. Her respondents experienced denial, anger, bargaining, depression, and, sometimes, eventual acceptance. As Kübler-Ross has noted, these siblings did not necessarily proceed through these stages in an orderly or unidirectional fashion. Titleman and Psyk (1991) provided further support for the experience of mourning in siblings. In their work they were able to identify as common experiences profound sadness, guilt, unconscious identification with the sibling suffering from schizophrenia, externalization of aspects of the survivor dilemma, and identification with a devastated and guilt-ridden parent.

It appears, then, that various patterns of response by siblings to mental illness have been identified in the literature. At one extreme, one can find attempts to rescue the ill relative. At the other, there is profound emotional and geographical separation from the disturbed sibling. Many alternate between disengagement and periodic attempts at intense involvement with the patient, family, and/or treatment team. While it must be recognized that this does not apply to all, the literature supports the contention that many siblings are at risk. For example, Johnson (1988) contrasts the overinvolved, self-neglectful caretaker with the sibling who is totally removed from the situation, and who may utilize disengagement as a general life strategy. Others reported that the majority of well siblings who were involved in family interaction were functioning poorly and developed personal difficulties. Conversely, some developed rigid boundaries which isolated them from the family turmoil. This latter group of siblings tended to live a relatively safe but constricted existence (Hoover & Franz, 1972).

*Programs for Siblings*

Following on the growing interest and awareness on the part of mental health professionals, specific kinds of interventions have been proposed for siblings. Since siblings are not a single homogeneous population, and the issues they face are both complex and varied, a broad spectrum of programs has been suggested.

Landeen and colleagues (1992) advocate for a sibling-oriented psycho-educational approach similar to well-established programs for families (Anderson, Reiss, & Hogarty, 1986; Bernheim & Lehman, 1985). She argues that such a program should include specific content addressing the information needs of the siblings as well as providing an opportunity for sharing experiences with others. This approach seems geared to those siblings who are less immediately involved in the care of their ill relative and perhaps worried about overinvolvement with helping professionals, but are willing to learn more about the illness without making a commitment to treatment. For those who have more direct involvement or want help with personal distress related to the patient's illness, this approach could be used as an adjunct to other interventions.

Other clinicians have advocated for the inclusion of siblings in family therapy (Vandereycken & Van Vreckem, 1992; Roberto, 1988). Harris (1988), for example, included siblings with their parents and the patient in family therapy and attempted to change rigid, constricted role enactments, and thus make room for the needs of other family members, including those of the siblings. He also offered and continues to provide sibling groups with a more expressive focus. As discussed earlier, many of the authors offer individual psychotherapy or psychoanalysis for those who are interested in a more intensive treatment wherein they can examine the meaning of their sibling relationship and the illness (Titleman & Psyk, 1991; Bank & Kahn, 1982; Graham, 1988).

One other approach seeks to help siblings and other caregivers achieve balance and control in their lives to enhance the capacity to choose alternatives on the basis of practicality balanced with the acceptability of their consequences (Johnson, 1988). Johnson advocates the use of self-help groups oriented to an eight-stage process to support the working-through of some of the principal emotional issues to achieve a changed view of self and of the relationship to the patient and others. Johnson (1988) has been instrumental in the development of the National Sibling Network, which organizes groups and publishes a quarterly newsletter, *The Sibling Bond*, with circulation throughout the United States.

## Summary

Our knowledge about the siblings of the mentally ill remains limited. The recent increase in interest in the experience of siblings is promising. However, we do not yet have an integrated theoretical framework and supportive empirical data to guide our work. Many areas remain poorly understood or unexplored. The few studies which have directly asked siblings what they need and want (Landeen et al., 1992; Riebschleger, 1991) have offered different results. Despite these shortcomings, there is some direction regarding the most important questions to address with siblings. First, and foremost, is: Are siblings affected by psychiatric disorder in a brother or sister? The answer appears to be broadly, yes. The effects seem to vary in significance and visibility with the degree of involvement with the patient, the pre-existing relationship, family dynamics and constellation, and the patient's acceptance of and the outcome of treatment. The impact of the illness tends to be far reaching and there are complex tasks associated with mourning the loss of a 'normal' sibling. Another question is: Are siblings harmed by this experience? The answer, at best, is, perhaps. An unknown number develop significant disturbances like those discussed by the early investigators (Lidz et al., 1963; Meissner, 1970). What differentiates siblings at risk for significant disturbance from those who remain resilient? The literature certainly provides some answers, but they are far from complete. Presumably Bank and Kahn are correct when they suggest that the age and developmental stage of the sibling, the rate of onset and chronicity of illness, and the degree of embarrassment brought on by the symptoms affect the degree of burden experienced. A strong family or other support network for both patient and sibling seems to make a difference, as do other demands in the sibling's life. Another dimension is added by Bank and Kahn's concept of the 'sibling bond' and by Graham's notion of a separate sibling separation–individuation developmental line. These intricate and complex processes are deeply embedded in the psychological and emotional make-up of the individual and may culminate in a close affectionate bond, one that is distant and hostile, a more balanced one, or merely a connection with someone who is not known well and with whom there is little relationship. Similarly, while Riebschleger's informants, and 'first-person' authors such as Aronowitz and Brodoff, are not disturbed, their distress is painful and significant. The intrusion of the illness may thrust the sibling into a position diametrically opposed to the one which the natural unfolding of these processes had decreed. Thus, there may be great anger towards a sibling once loved and admired, a sense of obligation towards one who was disowned or who was of marginal importance.

For those siblings with some level of involvement in the patient's care, the question arises as to how much they are able to manage. The nature of parental involvement is presumably an influence. If a sibling is the sole caretaker, the question assumes even greater urgency. The prevailing wisdom with respect to children has been that a sibling who is sole caretaker without significant adult support cannot effectively take the place of a parent (Bank and Kahn, 1982). However, adults, even psychiatrically ill adults, are not children, and adult siblings may have achieved sufficient maturity and personal stability to enable them to do more. The authors differ on what is possible. Bank & Kahn (1982) state that 'for most people it is impossible to do a job well and care for home, children, spouse and for a chronically ill sibling' (p. 262). They believe that siblings can be effective caregivers over a relatively short period of time when their identification remains partial, so that they are engaged but objective. Additionally, these authors have suggested that effective sibling involvement is much less likely when symptoms are protracted, dangerous, or embarrassing. Conversely, Johnson (1988) has argued that 'you can choose to be a caregiver – to enjoy your life and all your relationships ... the choice is yours, escaping or living ... someone else's behaviour doesn't cause you to be unhappy, it is your response to this behaviour' (p. 41). Either of these positions might be correct in a given situation, although it must be said that Johnson's level of optimism seems to be somewhat excessive.

In the light of this complexity, the range of programs and interventions that have been proposed makes intuitive sense as they can be used as links in a sensitive, comprehensive system of response to a spectrum of highly diverse needs. Ideally, the full range of programs suggested would potentially be available to any sibling, and offered according to individual need. Siblings can benefit from increased sensitivity to these issues so that they will be acknowledged, appropriately included, and no longer left silent and forgotten.

REFERENCES

Abarbanel, J. (1983). The revival of the sibling experience during the mother's second pregnancy. *Psychoanalytic Study of the Child, 38*, 353–379.

Anderson, C.M., Reiss, D.J., & Hogarty, G.E. (1986). *Schizophrenia and the family: A practitioner's guide to psychoeducation and management.* New York: Guilford.

Aronowitz, P. (1988, 24 January). A brother's dreams. *New York Times Magazine,* p. 35.

Bernheim, K.F., & Lehman, A.F. (1985). *Working with families of the mentally ill.* New York: W.W. Norton.

Bank, S.P., & Kahn, M.D. (1982). *The sibling bond.* New York: Basic Books.

Brodoff, A.S. (1988). First person account: Schizophrenia through a sister's eyes – The burden of invisible baggage. *Schizophrenia Bulletin, 14,* 113–116.

Colonna, A.B., & Newman, L.M. (1983). The psychoanalytic literature on siblings. *The Psychoanalytic Study of the Child, 38,* 285–309.

Dunn, J. (1992). Sister and brothers: Current issues in developmental research. In F. Boer and J. Dunn (Eds.), *Children's sibling relationships: Developmental and clinical issues* (pp. 1–18). Hillsdale, NJ: Lawrence Erlbaum Associates.

Dunn, J., & Plomin, R. (1991). Why are siblings so different? The significance of differences in sibling experiences within the family. *Family Process, 30,* 271–283.

Goetting, A. (1986). The developmental tasks of siblingship over the life cycle. *Journal of Marriage and the Family, 48,* 703–714.

Gold, D.T. (1989). Generational solidarity: Conceptual antecedents and consequences. *American Behavioural Scientist, 33* (1), 19–32.

Graham, I. (1988). The sibling objects and its transferences: Antecedents and consequences. *Psychoanalytic Inquiry, 8* (1), 88–107.

Harris, E.G. (1988). My brother's keeper: Siblings of chronic patients as allies in family treatment. In M.D. Kahn & K.G. Lewis (Eds.), *Siblings in therapy: Life span and clinical issues* (pp. 314–338). New York: W.W. Norton.

Hatfield, A.B. (1987). Families as caregivers: A historical perspective. In A.B. Hatfield & H.P. Lefley (Eds.), *Families of the mentally ill: Coping and adaptation* (pp. 3–29). New York: Guilford.

Hoover, C.F., & Franz, J.D. (1972). Siblings in the families of schizophrenics. *Archives of General Psychiatry, 26,* 334–342.

Jaffe, P. (1992). First person account: My brother. *Schizophrenia Bulletin, 18,* 155–156.

Johnson, J.T. (1988). *Hidden victims: An eight-stage healing process for families and friends of the mentally ill.* New York: Doubleday.

Kris, M., & Ritvo, S. (1983). Parents and siblings: Their mutual influences. *Psychoanalytic Study of the Child, 38,* 311–324.

Kübler-Ross, E. (1969). *On death and dying.* New York: Macmillan.

Landeen, J.L., Whelton, C.L., Dermer, S.W., Camardone, J., Munroe-Blum, H., & Thornton, J.F. (1992). Needs of well siblings of clients with schizophrenia. *Hospital and Community Psychiatry, 43,* 266–269.

Leitchman, M. (1985). The influence of an older sibling on the separation–individuation process. *Psychoanalytic Study of the Child, 40*, 111–161.

Lidz, T., Fleck, S., Alanen, Y.O., & Cornelison, A.R. (1963). Schizophrenic patients and their siblings. *Psychiatry, 26*, 1–18.

Meissner, W.W. (1970). Sibling relations in the schizophrenic family. *Family Process, 9*, 1–25.

Neubauer, P.B. (1983). The importance of the sibling experience. *Psychoanalytic Study of the Child, 38*, 325–336.

Newman, G. (1966). Younger brothers of schizophrenics. *Psychiatry, 29*, 146–151.

Provence, S., & Solnit, A.J. (1983). Development-promoting aspects of the sibling experience. *Psychoanalytic Study of the Child, 38*, 337–351.

Riebschleger, J.L. (1991). Families of chronically mentally ill people: Siblings speak to social workers. *Health and Social Work, 16*, 94–103.

Roberto, L.G. (1988). The vortex: Siblings in the eating disordered family. In M. Kahn & K. Lewis (Eds.), *Siblings in therapy: Life span and clinical issues* (pp. 297–313). New York: W.W. Norton.

Ross, H., & Milgram, J. (1982). Important variable in adult sibling relationships. In M. Lamb & B. Sutton-Smith (Eds.), *Sibling relationships: Their nature and significance across the life span* (pp. 223–247). Hillsdale, NJ: Lawrence Erlbaum Associates.

Samuels, L., & Chase L. (1979). The well siblings of schizophrenics. *The American Journal of Family Therapy, 7*, 24–35.

Simon, C. (1993, 18 July). The family madness. *Boston Globe.*

Thornton, J.F., Plummer, E., Seeman, M.V., & Littmann, S.K. (1981). Schizophrenia: Group support for relatives. *Canadian Journal of Psychiatry, 26*, 341–344.

Titelman, D., & Psyk, L. (1991). Grief, guilt, and identification in siblings of schizophrenic individuals. *Bulletin of the Menninger Clinic, 55*, 72–84.

Vandereycken, W., & Van Vreckem, E. (1992). Siblings as co-patients and co-therapists in eating disorders. In F. Boer & J. Dunn (Eds.), *Children's sibling relationships: Developmental and clinical issues* (pp. 109–124). Hillsdale, NJ: Lawrence Erlbaum Associates.

Waring, E.M., Carver, C., Moran, P., & Lefooe, D.H. (1986). Family therapy and schizophrenia: Recent developments. *Canadian Journal of Psychiatry, 31*, 154–160.

# The Impact of Parental Affective Disorders on Families

## TATYANA BARANKIN AND MYRNA GREENBERG

Affective disorders (major depression, bipolar affective disorder, and dysthymic disorders) are common conditions in the general population with a point prevalence of 9 to 20 per cent at any given time (Boyd & Weissman, 1981). They are recurrent and pervasive, and affect the overall functioning of the person and the family (Keller et al., 1983; Keller, 1988). These disorders are chronic in approximately 25 per cent of depressed patients, and 20 per cent fail to recover from an episode (Depue & Munroe, 1986). Affective disorders often affect women of child-bearing age and therefore potentially have a significant impact on early mother–child interactions (Radke-Yarrow et al., 1985; Cohn et al., 1990). Affective disorders are a common public health problem (see table 9.1).

The body of knowledge regarding the impact of parental affective disorders on children and the awareness of the importance of reducing the deleterious effects have been growing. Until recently, these issues en neglected, and those children at risk for affective disorders developmental difficulties have remained unidentified. Commu- rkers, public health nurses, social workers, and family doctors should play a pivotal role in early identification of these chil- risk.

dvances in psychopharmacology, more people are being treated -patient basis, and hospital stays have been reduced. Conse- hildren have more exposure to the symptoms of mental illness fewer separations from their parents. Unfortunately, both the s of the illness and the side-effects of some medication can, and , affect parental emotional availability.

ssay addresses the impact of parental affective disorder on the vith a particular focus on the children. Theoretical and clinical

Table 9.1
Affective Disorders Are a Major Public Health Problem

---

- Affective disorders are common: point prevalence 9 to 20 per cent
- Affective disorders are pervasive: they impair major life functions of the patient, and his or her spouse and children
- Affective disorders are recurrent: 50 to 85 per cent of unipolar patients seeking treatment experience additional episodes
- Affective disorders are chronic in 25 per cent of patients
- Affective disorders are increasingly more frequent, and age of onset is shifting downward
- Affective disorders lead to increased rate of divorce and family discord
- Children of parents with affective disorders have a threefold increase in psychopathology

---

issues are discussed, and a case example is presented to illustrate the importance of early identification and treatment of families at risk.

## The Nature/Nurture Debate

In an effort to evaluate the relative strength of genetic and environmental factors in the genesis of affective disorders, twin studies and studies of adopted individuals have been conducted. In Denmark, Bertelsen, Harvald, and Hauge (1977) studied 110 twin pairs in which at least one sibling suffered from a unipolar or bipolar disorder. The concordance rate for monozygotic twins was 0.67, whereas that for dizygotic pairs it was 0.20. Since monozygotic twins are said to share the same genetic information, and have the highest concordance rate, investigators have argued for a genetic basis for affective disorders. That is, the genes of affected persons have a vulnerability or propensity towards affective disorders. The fact that both bipolar disorders and unipolar depression run in families is also consistent with a biological cause for mood disorders (Kaplan & Sadock, 1991).

Adoption studies have attempted to clarify the respective contribution of genetic and family-related factors in the etiology of affective disorders (Cadoret et al., 1985; Mendewicz & Rainer, 1977; Knorring et al., 1983; Wender et al., 1985; Kety, Rosenthal, & Wender, 1971). An eightfold greater frequency of unipolar depression among the biological relatives of the depressed individuals compared with controls, and an increased rate of attempted and completed suicide and alcohol dependence in relatives of patients with a diagnosis of affective disorder and/or schizophrenia, have been reported (Wender et al., 1985).

In addition to the strong support for a biological cause for mood disorders, there is clear evidence that environmental factors also contribute to

Table 9.2

Characteristics of Family Environment in Families with Affective Illness

- Unpredictability and frequent chaos of the family environment
- Role reversal between parents and children
- Periods of relative or actual neglect
- Inconsistency of physical and psychological attention given towards children
- Hostility of depressed mother towards children
- Spouses are often mentally disturbed themselves, and marriage often deteriorates
- The 'well' spouse experiences role overload. If the 'well' spouse decompensates, the children lose the protective buffer against the ill parent's hostility or neglect

the impairment in offspring of the mentally ill. These include family dysfunction, lack of adequate external support systems (school, religious institutions, community), and poor socio-economic status (Keitner et al., 1986; Swindle, Cronkite, & Moos, 1989). A chaotic and disruptive family environment, periods of relative or actual neglect, and unpredictability and inconsistency in the caretaking environment have also been described as being potentially damaging (Guttman, 1989). The importance of a well- ─ functioning spouse or extended family is well documented and appears to buffer the pathogenic effect of the illness on the child (Fisher et al., 1987). Unfortunately, this is not always possible since well spouses are often deeply affected by the illness, and can become dysfunctional themselves (Coyne et al., 1987; Fadden, Bebbington, & Kuipers, 1987).

**Family Functioning in Families with Affective Disorders**

In families where one parent suffers from a mood disorder, family functioning is frequently characterized by unpredictability and chaos, periods of relative or actual neglect, role reversal between parents and children, marital discord, burn-out of the 'well' spouse, and inconsistency of physical and psychological attention given to children (see table 9.2). Most alarming is some evidence that the impaired family functioning one might expect during an acute phase of illness persists into and beyond the recovery period (Keitner & Miller, 1990).

*Family Functioning and the Phase of Depressive Illness*

During an acute depressive episode, women have been found to be more reticent in their communications, more submissive and dependent, less affectionate, and more argumentative with spouses and children (Weissman & Paykel, 1974). Greater levels of negative hostile behaviour, more self-preoccupation, negative tension, and more attempts at controlling other people have also been reported (Hinchliffe et al., 1975).

In 1985 Crowther studied family functioning in twenty-seven in-patients and compared the marital adjustment of those with major depression, schizophrenia, bipolar illness, and anxiety disorder. He reported that depressed patients had significantly more marital maladjustment than did the other patients with psychiatric illnesses. Furthermore, 40 per cent of adults living with a depressed patient were reported to have experienced a diagnosable psychiatric condition (Coyne et al., 1987).

Family functioning appears to improve as depression remits; however, families with affective illness still have more difficulty in communication and problem-solving when compared with non-clinical families (Keitner, Miller, & Epstein, 1987; Merikangas, Prusoff, & Kupfer, 1985). Current available data suggest that disturbed family functioning is associated with overall lower rates of recovery, and slower recovery among patients who do remit (Rounsaville, Weissman, & Prusoff, 1979; Corney, 1987; Keitner, Miller, & Epstein, 1987). Family functioning has also been found to influence rates of recovery and relapse. One concept that has received considerable attention in the literature is that of 'expressed emotion' (EE), a term that refers to critical comments and emotional overinvolvement by significant others.

It has been reported that depressed patients whose family members had a high level of 'expressed emotion' (EE) were three times as likely to relapse within nine months, when compared with those whose relatives had low levels of 'expressed emotion' (Vaughn & Leff, 1976; Hooley, Orley, & Teasdale, 1986).

Regardless of the interpretation, there is sufficient evidence which suggests that depression takes a tremendous toll on families, and one is left wondering about the impact of parental affective disorder on children. Specifically, are the children in these families more likely to develop psychiatric illnesses and/or have developmental difficulties?

A number of investigators have reported that there is a higher incidence of affective disorders in children of parents with major depression. The rate of disorders is 23 to 38 per cent in families with depression, compared with 11 to 24 per cent in control families (Weissman et al., 1984; Orvachel, Weissman, & Kidd, 1980; Orvachel, Walsh-Allis, & Ye, 1988; Cytryn et al., 1982; Weissman et al., 1987; Weissman et al., 1992). Weissman and colleagues (1984) reported both a threefold increase in psychiatric diagnoses in children of parents with an affective illness and an earlier onset of major depression in children of depressed parents.

In 1985, Akiskal and colleagues studied the juvenile offspring of patients with a manic-depressive illness. The study showed that approximately half of the sample displayed signs of bipolarity during a three-year prospective follow-up, and 40 per cent of the prepubertal children studied had hypomanic features. Extrapolating from these findings, Akiskal and colleagues estimated that bipolar spectrum disorders develop in about 27 per cent of children with one affected parent and suggested that the risk would be almost three times as high if both parents were ill. Like the children of depressed parents, the offspring of patients with manic-depressive illness were given several diagnoses, including major depression, dysthymic disorder, attention deficit disorder, separation anxiety, and conduct disorder.

Loss and separation from the caregiver, insecure and ambivalent attachments, introjected hostility, and impoverished and unstable caregiving environments have been associated with the development of depression in children of parents with a bipolar affective disorder (Anthony, 1975). These children were also found to have difficulty sharing with their friends and managing hostility, and had maladaptive patterns of aggression (Davenport et al., 1984; Gaensbauer et al., 1984; Zahn-Waxler et al., 1984). Interestingly, the social and emotional problems of these children are similar to the interpersonal problems reported by parents with manic-depressive illness. Parents with bipolar affective disorder have been described as persons who take but refuse to give, have little awareness of others as people, have little ability for empathy, and have a diminished capacity for fostering stable secure attachments in the child because of their own infantile dependency needs (Anthony, 1975). Parents with bipolar affective disorder have also been found to have difficulty mastering issues of loss, grief, and rage, and have developed defensive manoeuvres to avoid conflict. They also have problems initiating and sustaining intimacy with those outside their own family (Davenport et al., 1984). In light of these parallels, one wonders whether children develop problems with emotional regulation through modelling or whether these early dificulties are predictive of later onset of disease. The answer to this question remains unknown.

In addition to the problems with emotional regulation that are transmitted genetically or through modelling, a number of illness factors have been found to have a direct impact on child functioning and behaviour (see table 9.3). These include the severity and chronicity of the parental illness, the parent's insight into his or her condition, compliance with treatment, and co-morbidity. When a disorder is severe, with frequent

Table 9.3
Protective and Pathogenic Factors Affecting Adaptation
in Children of Mood-Disordered Parents

1. Factors Related to Parental Illness
   - diagnosis
   - comorbidity
   - chronicity
   - age of child at onset of parental illness

2. Factors Related to the Child
   - biological (I.Q.)
   - genetic (studying pedigree for loading)
   - temperament
   - general health
   - self-concept/competence
   - interpersonal relationships
   - relationship with well parent

3. Factors Related to Family Functioning
   - marital discord
   - communication style
   - expression of affect
   - availability of social support
   - socio-economic status

exacerbations, or where a personality disorder or alcoholism coexists and there is poor compliance or poor response to treatment, the impact on the family is more pronounced (Keller et al., 1986; Sameroff, Seifer, & Barocas, 1983). Chronicity and a narrow range of affective expression were also found to be associated with poorer child functioning (Wynne, Cole, & Perkins, 1987).

In summary, the better the marital adjustment, the better the child adjustment. Parental personality disorder and co-morbidity have deleterious effects. Generally, the more chronic the affective disorder, the poorer the prognosis for children. However, 'well' spouse adjustment to the illness enhances a child's ability to cope. Finally, there is a higher incidence of affective disorders and non-affective symptomatology in the offspring of parents with mood disorders.

## Invulnerability, Resilience, and Competence

Despite the high risk of psychopathology in the offspring of mentally ill parents, some children do emerge as energetic, well balanced, and resilient. The invulnerable child as described by Anthony (1974) has a seemingly stubborn resistance to the process of being engulfed by illness, develops a level of knowledge about the illness, and neither retreats from nor is intimidated by the problem. Instead, the child is able to view the illness as something needing to be understood.

Keller and colleagues (1986) found that 54 per cent of the children of parents with chronic affective disorder with psychotic features were generally happy and able to cope adequately with their problems, and that self-understanding significantly contributed to resilience. Self-esteem, mastery, autonomy, the capacity for flexibility, good coping strategies, parental supervision, a good stable relationship with an adult, the ability to exert control over one's environment, and attendance at good schools were also found to be important factors which enhance competence in children (El-Guebaly & Offord, 1980).

It appears that children with greater assets (intelligence, higher socio-economic status, and positive family attributes of stability and cohesion) are more competent and more socially connected (Garmezy, 1987; Garmezy & Bevine, 1984). According to Beardslee and Podorefsky (1988, p. 67), 'resilient' adolescents whose parents have serious affective disorders have been found to have:

1 Above average intelligence, no psychological distress, and no neurodevelopmental disabilities that could interfere with their ability to adapt to stress.
2 Resilient children demonstrated courage, motivation, and a strong sense of personal integrity.
3 There was a higher degree of self-understanding among invulnerable children.
4 They were aware of the parental illness and were realistic about the consequences of their own actions. Over time they accepted the fact that they could not cure their parents and did not assume responsibility for the illness.
5 Resilient children were able to think and act separately.

*Opportunities for Prevention*

Children of parents with affective disorders present a unique opportunity to mental health professionals for the early identification and prevention of the serious sequelae associated with psychiatric illness (see table 9.4).

Table 9.4
Prevention in Population at Risk for Affective Disorders

---

1. Primary Prevention
   Interventions designed to reduce a disorder in a target population:
   • genetic counselling
   • prevention of child neglect
2. Secondary Prevention
   Early identification and remediation of problem areas, which could include:
   • Early diagnosis of postpartum depression in mother with attention to mother–child attachment process and mother's attunement to child's needs
   • Early identification of a child at risk and prompt intervention
   • Regular annual check-up of children in families with psychiatric illness

3. Tertiary Prevention
   • Rehabilitation efforts to maximize the child's potential for normative experiences

---

Depression is a major mental illness with a high prevalence rate, particularly in women of child-bearing age. As well, the literature indicates that children of parents with affective disorders have 25 to 50 per cent rates of psychopathology. These statistics make these children and families ideal candidates for preventive treatment approaches. However, these opportunities are often overlooked (Phillips, 1983).

A number of opportunities exist for illness prevention in children. Improvement of family functioning, enhanced support for the well spouse and children, and early diagnosis and treatment of depression in the postpartum period are just a few of the possibilities (Laroche, 1986). The clinic for Children at Risk at the Clarke Institute of Psychiatry, in Toronto, Ontario, addresses secondary prevention and aims at identifying children at risk for affective disorders and/or developmental difficulties. It also treats youngsters who have diagnosable conditions. A cognitive psychoeducational approach, based on the work of Beardslee (1990), is used. Family strengths are identified, and there is a clear focus on the present and future needs of the children.

*Case History*

Although every family is unique, with its own complement of strengths and weaknesses, stresses, and coping strategies, families in which one parent suffers from a mood disorder share many of the same challenges and difficulties. A closer look at a particular family reveals many of those commonalities. Linda and Janice Stone are able to give a poignant account of their experiences growing up in a family in which their mother suffers from a mood disorder.

Linda, age seven, was born with a neurodegenerative disease. She is blind in one eye and has some difficulties with articulation. She is intelligent and gregarious, demanding attention from everyone around her. She says she worries a lot about her family, especially when her mother is ill. Her parents argue and Linda tries to get between them to stop the fighting. Linda says she and her sister are the saddest in the family because her parents argue so much. She has dreams which frighten her and make her sad. She tells Janice about her dreams but is afraid to tell her parents because she believes the dreams might then come true.

Nine-year-old Janice, thin, dark-haired, and pretty, appears more anxious and withdrawn than her sister, Linda. She is worried that the doctors will not find the right medicine for her mother and that she will be in hospital for a long time. Janice also worries that her father will not return when he goes away on business trips. She fears he may die.

In many ways, Janice is a parentified child. She comforts her sister and tries to help her. She vacuums and cleans the house when her mother is not well. She says she can turn to her father for comfort when she is sad or frightened, but often does not talk to him because she worries he will argue with her mother.

Janice has nightmares, which began after she saw her mother attempt suicide. Once, when Janice was sleepwalking, her father found her carrying a knife. She reluctantly describes a dream in which both of her parents died: A man came by and was able to bring her father back to life but was not able to save her mother. Janice is afraid to tell her mother about the dream because she worries her mother will think she loves her father more. Janice also worries about her sister's illness, but is careful not to talk about it in Linda's presence.

Both Linda and Janice notice a big difference at home when their mother is ill. They are not allowed to watch television or to go out as much. Linda says her mother stops making their favourite foods and they have to eat the same thing day after day.

The last time Mrs Stone was hospitalized, Linda and Janice had to change schools temporarily while they stayed with their grandmother. At times when Mrs Stone is depressed at home, she loses her patience with the children. Janice says her mother gets angry and shakes her. Mr Stone claims that at one point his wife bit Janice's leg.

Janice and Linda's maternal grandmother often helps out when her daughter is ill. Both girls are able to turn to her for support. Often, though, Janice does not talk to her because she is afraid her mother will think her grandmother is interfering. None the less, she often stays with her grandchildren when Mrs Stone is not well, making sure they get to school on time and have regular meals.

Janice says that, when her mother is better, she is fun to be with and makes her favourite foods. She allows Linda and Janice to have more freedom, and the family goes on outings together. Neither Linda nor Janice wants to talk about 'bad things' when their mother is better. They fear their mother will become ill again and that their parents will start to argue.

Mr and Mrs Stone, ages thirty-nine and thirty-five, respectively, have been married for ten years. They are a well-educated and attractive couple. Both agree that they began having marital problems seven years ago, but each identifies different reasons for the difficulties. There is little warmth between them and they barely speak to each other.

Mr Stone says he feels hopeless. He speaks with a quiet anger. He used to be more outgoing and to enjoy socializing. Since his wife became ill he has been more withdrawn. He blames Mrs Stone. He feels she denies that she has an illness and says she does not follow her doctor's directions. He counts her pills and accuses her of not taking her medication. He is angry because she makes decisions about the children without talking to him. He has been considering divorcing his wife. He told Mrs Stone that he will leave her if she does not take her medication.

Mr Stone worries about Janice, who has frequent colds and bites her fingernails. He thinks she is a nervous child. He is worried about her nightmares and sleepwalking, fearing she may hurt herself. He also worries about Linda. He feels helpless about her chronic illness.

Mrs Stone suffered from a depression following Linda's birth. She lost weight and was unable to sleep. She speaks quietly with long pauses between herthoughts. Her depressions are cyclical according to her husband, with ten good days and ten bad. For the most part, Mrs Stone's illness has not responded well to medication. It is difficult to determine the extent to which her adjusting her own medication has contributed to this problem. It is clear that, when Mrs Stone is not depressed, she is a warm and caring mother to her children.

Mrs Stone believes her depression is a reaction to her husband's behaviour towards her. She feels he is unsupportive and critical. She believes the children's difficulties stem from the conflict between herself and Mr Stone. She says she would like to attend marital counselling with her husband.

When Mrs Stone is free of depression, the family functions well, in spite of the chronic tension between herself and her husband. They are able to have fun together and enjoy each other.

Although several complicating factors enter into this family's situation, not the least of which is Mr and Mrs Stone's unresolved mourning of Linda's chronic illness, their experience is in many ways typical of that of families in which one parent suffers from a mood disorder.

There has been chronic marital discord since Mrs Stone became ill. Her hospitalizations lead to disruptions in the children's daily routines. What may perhaps be more disruptive for the children is dealing with Mrs Stone's depression when she is not in hospital. She can be controlling and intrusive, has limited patience, and has, on a least one occasion, been physically abusive. The marital conflict frightens the children and heightens their insecurity about the stability of their family. Mr Stone is depleted and angry much of the time, and this limits his ability to be responsive to his children's needs.

Both Linda and Janice expend a great deal of energy worrying about their mother's illness and the conflict between their parents. Janice has taken on a parenting role with her sister and this gets in the way of developing her own potential. The anxiety Linda and Janice are experiencing has begun to take a toll on their school work.

A significant protective factor for these children is their relationship with their grandmother. She helps out instrumentally when Mrs Stone is ill, as well as providing a reality base and sympathetic ear for the children. Both Janice and Linda are intelligent, open, and insightful. In spite of the adverse conditions affecting this family, the children have obviously benefited from considerable nurturing provided by both parents. Their strengths can be reinforced by therapy aimed at helping them cope more effectively with their fears and anxieties.

Treatment
The treatment plan for this family consisted of both parenting sessions and sibling sessions. Psychoeducational and problem-solving techniques were used to enable the parents to work together more effectively to meet their children's needs for predictability and consistency. Sibling therapy provided the children with a safe enviornment to express their fears and concerns; helped them to develop strategies to cope more effectively with their mother's illness and the conflict between their parents; and provided education about mood disorders to decrease their guilt about contributing to their mother's illness.

## Conclusions

As is evident from the theoretical and clinical review, children and families of parents with an affective illness experience significant emotional difficulties. Marital discord is very common and may contribute to a child's distress, and to relapse in the ill parent.

Biological, genetic, psychological, and social factors influence the development of psychopathology in the offspring and spouses of patients with mood disorders. The severity and chronicity of the illness, marital discord, and the presence of criticism and hostility in family communications have potentially deleterious effects on the child and can adversely affect family functioning. Despite these problems, approximately one-half of the children from families in which a parent has an affective disorder are able to grow up to become energetic, well-balanced individuals. Resilience in the face of adversity helps these children and families cope successfully with the multiple stressors of a mood disorder. Emerging data from the literature indicate that, because of the familial nature of mood disorders, treatment should include the family. Psychoeducational cognitive approaches conducted in the context of the family have proven to be particularly effective. Further research is needed to investigate the efficacy of currently available treatments with these families.

REFERENCES

Akiskal, M.S., Downs, J., Jordon, P., Watson, S., Dougherty, D., & Pruitt, D.B. (1985). Affective disorders in referred children and younger siblings of manic depressives. *Archives of General Psychiatry, 42*, 996–1003.
Anthony, E.J. (1974). The syndrome of the psychologically invulnerable child. In E.J. Anthony & A.E. Koypernic (Eds.), *The child in his family: Children at psychiatric risk* (pp. 529–544 ). New York: John Wiley.
Anthony, E.J. (1975). The influence of a manic-depressive environment on the developing child. In E.J. Anthony, and T. Beneden (Eds.), *Depression and human existence* (pp. 279–315). Boston: Little, Brown.
Beardslee, W.R. (1990). Development of a clinician-based preventive intervention for families with affective disorders. *Journal of Preventive Psychiatry and Allied Disciplines, 4* (1), 39–60.
Beardslee, W.R., & Podorefsky, D. (1988). Resilient adolescents whose parents have serious affective and other psychiatric disorder: Importance of self-understanding and relationships. *American Journal of Psychiatry, 145*, 63–69.

Bertelsen, A., Harvald, B., & Hauge, M. (1977). A Danish twin study of manic-depressive disorders. *British Journal of Psychiatry, 130*, 330–351.

Boyd, J.M., & Weissman, M.M. (1981). Epidemiology of affective disorders. *Archives of General Psychiatry, 38*, 1039–1046.

Cadoret, R.J., O'Gorman, T.W., Heywood, E., & Troughton, E. (1985). Genetic and environmental factors in major depression. *Journal of Affective Disorders, 9*, 155–164.

Cohn, J.J., Campbell, S.B., Matias, R., & Hopkins, J. (1990). Face-to-face interactions of post-partum depressed and nondepressed mother–infant pairs at two months. *Developmental Psychology, 26* (1), 15–23.

Corney, R.M. (1987). Marital problems and treatment outcome in depressed women. *British Journal of Psychiatry, 151*, 652–659.

Coyne, J.C., Kessler, R.C., Tal, M., Turnbull, J., Wortman, C.G., & Greden, J. (1987). Living with a depressed person. *Journal of Consulting and Clinical Psychology, 55*, 347–352.

Crowther, J.H. (1985). The relationship between depression and marital maladjustment: A descriptive study. *Journal of Mental and Nervous Disease, 173*, 227–231.

Cytryn, E.M., McKnew, D., Bartko, J.J., Lamour, M., & Hamovit, J. (1982). Offspring of patients with affective disorder. *Journal of American Academy of Child Psychiatry, 21*, 389–391.

Davenport, Y., Zahn-Waxler, C., Adland, M., & Mayfield, A. (1984). Early child-rearing practices in families with a manic-depressive parent. *American Journal of Psychiatry, 141* (2), 230–235.

Depue, R.A., & Munroe, S.M. (1986). Conceptualization and measurement of human disorder and life stress research: The problem of chronic disturbance. *Psychological Bulletin, 99*, 36–51.

El-Guebaly, N., & Offord, D.R. (1980). The competent offspring of psychiatrically ill parents. *Canadian Journal of Psychiatry, 25*, 457–463.

Fadden, G., Bebbington, P., & Kuipers, L. (1987). Caring and its burdens: A study of the spouses of depressed patients. *British Journal of Psychiatry, 151*, 600–667.

Fisher, L., Kokes, R.F., Cole, R.E., Perkins, P.M., & Wynne, L.D. (1987). Competent children at risk: A study of well-functioning offspring of disturbed parents. In E.J. Anthony & B.J. Cohler (Eds.), *The invulnerable child* (pp. 211–228). New York: Guilford.

Gaensbauer, J.J., Harmon, R.J., Cytryn, L., & McKnew, D.M. (1984). Social and affective development in infants with a manic depressive parent. *American Journal of Psychiatry, 141*, 223–229.

Garmezy, N. (1987). Stress, competence and development. *American Journal of Orthopsychiatry, 57* (2), 159–174.

Garmezy, N., & Bevine, V. (1984). Project competence: The Minnesota studies of children vulnerable to psychopathology. In H. Watt, E.J. Anthony, L. Wynne, & S.J. Rolf (Eds.), *Children at risk for schizophrenia* (pp. 289–303). New York: Cambridge University Press.

Guttman, H.A. (1989). Children in families with emotionally disturbed parents. In L. Combrinck-Graham (Ed.), *Children in family contexts* (pp. 252–276). New York: Guilford.

Hinchliffe, M., Hooper, D., Roberts, F.J., & Vaughan, P.W. (1975). A study of the interaction between depressed patients and their spouses. *British Journal of Psychiatry, 126,* 164–172.

Hooley, J.M., Orley, J., & Teasdale, J.D. (1986). Levels of expressed emotions and relapse in depressed patients. *British Journal of Psychiatry, 148,* 642–647.

Kaplan, H., & Sadock, B. (1991). *Synopsis of psychiatry* ( 6th ed. ). London: Williams & Wilkins.

Keitner, G.I., & Miller, I.W. (1990). Family functioning and major depression: An overview. *American Journal of Psychiatry, 147* (9), 1128–1137.

Keitner, G.I., Miller, I.W., Epstein, N.B., & Bishop, D.S. (1986). The functioning of families of patients with major depression. *International Journal of Family Psychiatry, 7,* 11–16.

Keitner, G.I., Miller, I.W., & Epstein, N.B. (1987). Family functioning and the course of major depression. *Comprehensive Psychiatry, 28,* 54–64.

Keller, M.B. (1988). Diagnostic issues and clinical course of unipolar illness. In A.J. Frances & S.R.E. Hales (Eds.), *Review of psychiatry* (pp. 188–212). Washington, DC: American Psychiatric Press.

Keller, M.B., Lavori, P.W., Endicott, J., Coryell, W., & Klerman, G.L. (1983). Double depression: Two-year follow-up. *American Journal of Psychiatry, 140,* 689–694.

Keller, M.B., Beardslee, W.R., Dorer, D.J., Lavori, P.W., Samuelson, M., & Klerman, G.R. (1986). Impact of severity and chronicity of parental affective illness on adaptive functioning and psychopathology in children. *Archives of General Psychiatry, 43,* 930–937.

Kety, S.S., Rosenthal, D., & Wender, P.M. (1971). Mental illness in the biological and adoptive families of adopted schizophrenics. *American Journal of Psychiatry, 138,* 302–306.

Knorring, A.L., Von Cloninger, R., Bohman, M., & Sigvardsson, S. (1983). An adoption study of depressive disorders and substance abuse. *Archives of General Psychiatry, 40,* 943–950.

Laroche, C. (1986). Prevention in high risk children of depressed parents. *Canadian Journal of Psychiatry, 31,* 161–165.

Mendewicz, J., & Rainer, J.D. (1977). Adoption study supporting genetic transmission in manic-depressive illness. *Nature, 268,* 327–329.

Merikangas, K.P., Prusoff, B.A., & Kupfer, D.J. (1985). Marital adjustment in major depression. *Journal of Affective Disorders, 9,* 5–11.

Orvachel, H., Walsh-Allis, G., & Ye, W. (1988). Psychopathology in children of parents with recurring depression. *Journal of Abnormal Child Psychology, 16* (1), 17–28.

Orvachel, H., Weissman, M.M., & Kidd, K.V. (1980). Children and depression. *Journal of Affective Disorders, 2,* 1–16.

Phillips, I. (1983). Opportunities for prevention in the practice of psychiatry. *American Journal of Psychiatry, 140,* 389–395.

Radke-Yarrow, M., Cummings, E.M., Kuczynski, L., & Chapman, M. (1985). Patterns of attachment in two- and three-year-olds in normal families and families with paternal depression. *Child Development, 56,* 884–898.

Rounsaville, B.J., Weissman, M.M., & Prusoff, B.A. (1979). Marital disputes and treatment outcome in depressed women. *Comprehensive Psychiatry, 20,* 483–490.

Sameroff, A., Seifer, R., & Barocas, R. (1983). Impact of parental psychopathology: Diagnosis, severity, or social status effects? *Infant Mental Health Journal, 4* (3), 236–250.

Swindle, R.W., Jr, Cronkite, R.C., & Moos, R.M. (1989). Life stressors, social resources, coping, and the four-year course of unipolar depression. *Journal of Abnormal Psychology, 98,* 468–477.

Vaughn, C.F., & Leff, J.P. (1976). The influence of family and social factors on the course of psychiatric illness. *British Journal of Psychiatry, 129,* 125–137.

Weissman, M.M., Fendrich, M., Warner, V., & Wickramaratne, P. (1992). Incidence of psychiatric disorder in offspring at high and low risk for depression. *Journal of the American Academy of Child Psychiatry, 31* (4), 640–648.

Weissman, M.M., Gammon, D., John, K., & Merikangas, K.P. (1987). Children of depressed parents. *Archives of General Psychiatry, 44,* 847–853.

Weissman, M.M., & Paykel, E.S. (1974). *The depressed woman: A study of social relationships.* Chicago: University of Chicago Press.

Weissman, M.M., Prusoff, B.A., Gammon, G.D., Merikangas, K.R., Leckman, J.F., & Kidd, K.K. (1984). Psychopathology in the children (age 6–10) of depressed and normal parents. *Journal of the American Academy of Child Psychiatry, 23,* 78–84.

Wender, P.M., Kety, S.S., Rosenthal, D., Schulsinger, F., Ortmann, J., & Lunde, I. (1985). Psychiatric disorders in the biological and adoptive families of adopted individuals with affective disorders. *Archives of General Psychiatry, 43,* 923–929.

Wynne, L., Cole, R., & Perkins, P. (1987). University of Rochester child and family study: Risk research in progress. *Schizophrenia Bulletin, 13,* 403–476.

Zahn-Waxler, C., McKnew, D.M., Cummings, E.M., Davenport, Y.B., & Radke-Yarrow, M. (1984). Problem behaviors and peer interaction of young children with a manic-depressive parent. *American Journal of Psychiatry, 141,* 236–240.

# Mental Illness and Parenting Capacity: Assessing for Risk and Planning for Children

## CHRISTINA BARTHA AND LUIS GONCALVES

The field of child protection is challenging, given the difficult situations facing mental health professionals. In recent years, the law has shifted to provide parents every opportunity to care for their children before the termination of these rights is considered. This legal stipulation can present a particular dilemma to mental health professionals in situations where parents' functioning is marginal and it is unclear whether they can provide for their children's physical and emotional needs. Parents suffering from a mental illness present a unique challenge for clinicians. While — a diagnosis in itself does not determine parenting capacity, the symptoms can affect the caretaking skills and judgment of the parent. Assessing the impact of mental illness on parenting capacity requires the objective and systematic examination of functioning in a number of key areas.

Clinicians who conduct assessments of parents involved in disputes with child welfare authorities have struggled with the issues related to these cases. This essay highlights the literature which has contributed to knowledge in the field and presents a case application of the Toronto Parenting Capacity Assessment Project guidelines, an instrument designed to assist in assessing parenting skills. As well, several controversies which have arisen while working with this population of families are discussed.

Clinical approaches to the assessment of parenting capacity have been developed from a wide range of literature, including that covering the areas of child attachment, child development, and child psychopathology, as well as the study of the parent–child relationship. Within these areas, several researchers have focused exclusively on the children of parents with schizophrenia (Sameroff, Barocas, & Seifer, 1984; Weintraub, 1987), depression (Keller et al., 1986), and bipolar affective disorder (Laroche et al., 1987). Most 'at risk' are the children of parents with schizophrenia, approximately 50 per cent of whom will be maladjusted in adulthood and whose risk of developing the illness is ten to sixteen times greater than that of the general population (see Rosenthal, 1970, as cited by Weintraub, 1987). Offspring of depressed mothers are two to three times more at risk of developing a depressive disorder (Weissman & Boyd, 1985), and approximately 26 per cent of children of parents with a bipolar diagnosis may develop a depression of the dysthymic type (Laroche et al., 1987).

Many children enter the child welfare system as a result of their parents' mental health difficulties. Often, child protection workers are required to assess the parents' level of functioning and the degree of risk to the child. In these instances, understanding the impact of mental illness on parental functioning becomes an integral part of an assessment. Rather than provide a comprehensive review of the literature, which is beyond the scope of this essay, we highlight the work of several researchers and clinicians who have contributed to this field.

In the field of mental illness and parenting, research has developed in three main areas. Early findings established an unusually high rate of maladjustment among offspring whose parent or parents suffered from a major mental illness (Dodge, 1990). Some investigators examined the genetic transmission of mental illness from parents to offspring. However, given the large numbers of patients with no family history of illness, researchers soon considered the influences of environmental factors, such as family dynamics and poverty (ibid.). More recently, studies have examined parenting behaviours and their subsequent effect on child adjustment (Goodman & Brumley, 1990).

While results have been variable, in general, children of the mentally ill do more poorly on all measures of adjustment than do children of parents who are not ill (Seifer & Sameroff, 1981). All children of parents with a major psychiatric diagnosis fare even worse when they have also been exposed to unstable, unsatisfactory parenting (Weintraub, 1987). The offspring of the mentally ill who have fared most poorly are the children of parents with schizophrenia (Goodman & Brumley, 1990). The adjustment of children of parents with affective disorders has been found to be more variable: some present at least as poorly as children whose parents suffer from schizophrenia (Seifer & Sameroff, 1981), while others present more favourably (Goodman & Brumley, 1990).

Several researchers have focused on the social and intellectual development of these youngsters. Studies have found that children may withdraw from social interactions, deeming them unrewarding; show evidence of deficiencies in the development of social skills; or engage in coercive exchanges in a persistent effort to elicit the desired parental response (Cicchetti, 1987; Patterson, 1982; and Rubin, 1987, as cited by Goodman & Brumley, 1990). These children may be more self-critical and less self-rewarding. When their parents were less interested and more negative, they also displayed poorer intellectual functioning (Goodman & Brumley, 1990).

While some investigators have focused on maladjustment in these children, others have worked to identify those protective factors which allow children to develop without serious adjustment problems. These are of particular importance when assessing and planning for children living with disturbed parents. Werner and Smith (1982) conducted a longitudinal study which found several indicators that contribute to better adjustment, including more than one caretaker; a healthy or non-disturbed parent who was available to support the disturbed parent and model appropriate behaviour for the child; later onset of the parent's illness; fewer siblings in the family; and fewer recurring episodes of illness in the parent. Weintraub (1987) also found that children exposed to brief episodes of their parent's illness fared better than those who were exposed to chronic illness in the primary caretaker. In general, these factors clearly point to the need for a stable support system for the children, and protection from isolation with the ill parent. Often, this is accomplished by the involvement of extended family or the parent's partner. Assessing the skills and coping abilities of these supports may be important, particularly since the rate of marital conflict and breakdown remains quite high among the mentally ill (Hafner, 1986).

Recently, investigators have also focused on an interactional perspective which examines the impact of parenting style on children's adjustment, and considers the temperament and special needs of each child. Quality of parenting, rather than diagnosis, has been found to exert a greater influence on children's intellectual and social functioning (Goodman & Brumley, 1990). Mental illness can effect the ability of a parent to perceive and respond to a child's needs (Steinhauer, 1991). Parents suffering from schizophrenia may be withdrawn or emotionally unavailable to their children and may incorporate them into their delusions; children may also be exposed to their incongruent affect. Depressed parents may be emotionally unavailable and feel negatively towards their children. In general, it is the parents' lack of emotional involvement which has been found to have the most negative influence on the children's adjustment (Goodman & Brumley, 1990). In addition, parents' inattentiveness may explain the very high rate of childhood accidents which occur in these families (Gelfand &

Teti, 1990). Finally, environmental stressors, such as poverty and marital discord, have been found to have a negative effect on the parenting skills of this population, and to exacerbate problems (Weintraub, 1987; Goodman & Brumley, 1990). Interestingly, Goodman and Brumley (1990) found that the parenting skills of depressed mothers were not significantly poorer than those of single, impoverished mothers. This finding highlights the importance of considering the influence of environmental factors, such as poverty, on parenting.

While results to date provide important insights into the functioning of these families, further studies are needed as methodological shortcomings limit the degree to which one can generalize and compare findings (Rutter, 1990). Problems with previous studies include insufficient sample sizes, and homogenous samples which do not reflect the diverse socioeconomic and cultural nature of many communities. Despite the significant impact of poverty and maltreatment on family functioning and child adjustment, some studies have not controlled for these effects. This is highlighted by the study of Walker, Downey, and Bergman (1989), which found that children exposed to maltreatment were more aggressive and delinquent than those who were not: children who were exposed to maltreatment and a parent with schizophrenia fared even worse. Maltreatment, rather than parental diagnosis, was found to be a stronger predictor of poor child adjustment.

In some instances, when children are placed in care as a result of child protection concerns, visitation becomes the critical clinical issue. Few studies have addressed the impact of visitation on the parent–child relationship after children are placed in long-term foster care. This is an important issue when children cannot return to the custody of their parents but have established a significant attachment to them. Barnum (1987) and Steinhauer (1991) have noted that it may often be observed that children are resistant to visiting with natural parents. It is important that the reasons for such resistance be carefully assessed, as it may relate to a number of different factors, only one of which is the child's feelings towards the parent. Children may be torn between foster and natural parents, or observe hostile feelings which exist between the adults and professionals involved in the situation. Steinhauer (1991) cites several important reasons for maintaining visits between children and natural parents. These include:

**1. Visits to avoid agency- or court-created abandonment.** Children need to be reminded of their biological attachments; older children will likely recontact or return to their family of origin; thus, some ongoing connection should be maintained.

**2. Visits to catalyse the work of mourning.** Children seek to avoid the work of mourning the loss of their parents; these repressed feelings may be displaced onto foster parents, teachers, and others. Visits allow the child to re-experience these feelings, talk about them, and resolve what he or she has experienced. Visits with key people also help a child establish a sense of historical continuity and coherence. It is not the visits themselves, but how they are utilized to release the child's feelings and correct his or her perceptions of the natural family, which can assist potential resolution.

**3. The use of visits to undermine idealization of natural parents to whom a strong but negative bonding exists.** An older child who has no contact with natural parents may idealize the absent parent, thus alienating him- or herself even farther from current caretakers. Visits allow the child to experience the contrast between his or her fantasy and the reality of the natural parent, thus assisting the child in understanding why he or she is in care. As with the previous item, it is how the visits are used towards emotional resolution for the child which is of most importance.

Finally, Steinhauer (1991, p. 181) cited reasons for terminating contact between children and parents. He noted the real issue behind decisions around visits is 'the degree to which the child faces and deals successfully with both the facts and the associated feelings and fantasies of his life history.' Some children who have experienced severe abuse or neglect may not benefit from ongoing visits. Some parents may be unable to behave appropriately during visits, with the result that children are subjected to further rejection or criticism. Even in these situations, however, those children who state a wish not to see their parents should be followed-up from time to time to determine if their feelings have shifted to a desire for some contact. With other children, visits may perpetuate their reconciliation fantasies. These children may require a break in contact from natural parents in order to be free to form a meaningful attachment to their foster parents.

**Assessing for Parenting Capacity**

The clinical issue of whether to separate a child from his or her natural family has been fraught with controversy. Attempts to ensure that the best interests of children are of foremost concern and to prevent serious developmental damage may result in clinical dilemmas. Does one risk leaving the child in a marginal parenting situation in order to provide the parent every opportunity to improve, or does one risk permanently removing the child, which, in the long run, may be equally detrimental (Steinhauer, 1991)?

In 1989, the Toronto Parenting Assessment Project began to address this clinical question. The project is comprised of a multidisciplinary team of mental health professionals who have combined theoretical knowledge and clinical experience in developing a series of guidelines to be used when assessing parenting. The project team includes representatives from two local Children's Aid Societies, the Hospital for Sick Children, and the Family Court Clinic of Toronto.

The project has developed a clinical tool of nine comprehensive guidelines, which assists in the evaluation of current parenting ability and enables clinicians to predict future parenting capacity. Through the use of specific questionnaires, the clinician gathers the information required to make a sound clinical judgment. Although the criteria may be clear, the clinical judgments required are at best semi-objective, given the dependency on the assessor's skills, values, and biases. At the time of writing, the project was completing plans for field trials towards validating the guidelines. The dimensions are divided into four areas of focus, as outlined in table 10.1. All parameters are important, and to some extent interdependent. However, some dimensions may become more critical, given the clinical needs of a particular situation – for example, when a parent suffers from a mental illness.

The following is a brief summary of the clinical content that each guideline addresses.

**Guideline 1: Current Stressors.** It is important to understand the contextual stressors affecting parenting by conducting a social-environmental scan of: cultural or recent immigration status; housing conditions; poverty; unemployment; legal problems; history of violence or criminality; and severe or chronic illness in any family member.

**Guideline 2: Child's Developmental Progress.** A developmental delay may be a major indicator of parental neglect, especially with infants and younger children. It is necessary to conduct a developmental assessment of a child to assist in determining those select cases where more formal

Table 10.1
Guidelines for Assessing Parenting Capacity

---

A. Focus on the context
   Guideline 1. Current stressors

B. Focus on the child
   Guideline 2. Child's developmental progress

C. Focus on parent–child interrelationships
   Guideline 3. Predominant pattern of the child's response to caregiver
   Guideline 4. Observation of current parenting ability

D. Focus on the parent
   Guideline 5. Impulse control
   Guideline 6. Parental acceptance of responsibility
   Guideline 7. Problem behaviours affecting parenting ability and capacity
   Guideline 8. Parent's manner of relating to society
   Guideline 9. Parent's use of clinical interventions

---

developmental testing by a multidisciplinary team is indicated. This provides a baseline of a child's functioning against which further assessments could be compared, particularly in situations where there may be some doubt about the parent's influence on the child's progress.

**Guideline 3: Predominant Pattern of the Child's Response to Caregiver.** Understanding the nature of the child's attachment to the parent, and feelings of belonging, separation, and loss, is critical. Observations of the parent–child interactions should focus on the following: the child's preferences in contact with adults, including the assessor; whether a younger child plays independently and rarely checks in with the parent; and whether the child is distressed by a separation from the parent and is easily comforted upon the parent's return. It is also important to note whether the child behaves differently with other significant adults as compared with the biological parent. The assessor should list a history of the child's separations from the parent and inquire about the parent's own early parenting, and how he or she believes that experience influences his or her ability to meet the child's needs.

**Guideline 4: Observation of Current Parenting Ability.** Along with understanding the child's responses, it is equally important to assess the parental responses to the child, includeing: the parent's overall emotional availability: appropriateness of expectations; andeffectiveness and constructiveness of limit-setting. Observable behaviours to consider when assessing the parent's responses include: capacity to meet the child's basic needs; parental affective response and involvement; appropriateness of roles; disposition towards the child; ability to experience the child as separate; and management of the child.

**Guideline 5: Impulse Control.** Assessing the parent's ability to contain tension and negotiate a solution to problems, rather than frequently having explosive episodes, is particularly important, given a child's unpredictability and waywardness. The assessor should determine whether the parent is likely to approach stressful situations with an adequate measure of tolerance, rather than explosiveness, and whether the parent is habitually surrounded by tension-inducing or -reducing personal relationships which influence his or her parenting.

**Guideline 6: Parental Acceptance of Responsibility.** Assessing a person's ability to accept responsibility can be a subtle yet important task. The ability to reflect on one's own behaviour and accept one's shortcomings is an essential parenting skill. Is the parent able to assume responsibility for his or her behaviour rather than focus on blaming outside influences, such as relatives, agencies, or partners, for past or ongoing difficulties? Does the parent tend to consider the feelings of others or dismiss them? And, finally, is the parent primarily focused on his or her own feelings of rejection and discomfort?

**Guideline 7: Problem Behaviours Affecting Parenting Ability and Capacity.** When an individual suffers from a mental illness, the symptoms should be noted, as well as a description of their effect on parental functioning. It is important to distinguish between chronic or acute effects and how the behaviours affect the children in their day-to-day functioning. The major symptom areas of inquiry should include: depression; unstable mood; anxiety; poorly controlled rage, including verbal and physical violence; extreme perfectionism or constant criticism; ongoing substance abuse; delusions or hallucinations and/or a belief of persecution by others; defective judgment, such as extreme indecision; and apparent lack of intellectual ability.

**Guideline 8: Parent's Manner of Relating to Society.** How a parent generally relates with society may be similar to or different from his or her parenting style. It is important to establish whether there is a history of criminality or violence, apart from violence in the home. This assessment includes considering the availability and ability of the parent to use social and community supports by charting the parent's history of relating to social agencies, school systems, and other authority institutions in the community.

**Guideline 9: Parent's Use of Clinical Interventions.** Often families and individuals are or have been involved with various agencies and service providers. They may have undergone extensive assessments resulting in treatment recommendations. Understanding the parent's view and use of the clinical services, and identifying whether recommendations were followed-through provides insight into the parent's ability to form a therapeutic alliance. It is especially important to identify those services which the parent described as adequate, yet did not attend, as this is an indicator that the client will be even more difficult to engage in a helping relationship.

The use of these guidelines ensures a comprehensive assessment prior to professional decision making. It not only focuses on areas of concern, but considers strengths that may not be immediately apparent when working with parents who suffer from various types of impairment, including mental illness. It also provides a framework within which the clinician's biases and transferential issues can be monitored and addressed.

*Case History*

Child welfare cases are referred for assessment to the Family Court Clinic to assist the court in determining whether children in foster care should be returned to the custody of their parents, made wards of the state, or placed for adoption. In order to arrive at clinical recommendations, clinicians spend three to six months working with the parents and children. In addition to clinical interviews and observations, information from community agencies, such as child welfare authorities, physicians, and schools, is reviewed. When appropriate, clinicians work with parents on their parenting skills in order to determine their capacity to learn and retain new skills. This may be accomplished through individual parenting sessions or parent–child sessions.

Ms S. is the twenty-six-year-old mother of Jane (age seven), Tony (age three), and Tara (age one). Ms S. was from Hong Kong and had a family history of instability, and possible physical and sexual abuse. The children had been in foster care for one year since the onset of their mother's illness. The youngest child had been placed separately from her older brother and sister, who remained in the same foster home.

Until Jane was age five and Tony age one, Ms S. had successfully parented the children. Ms S. began to suffer from paranoid symptoms, believing that people were listening to her on the phone and at the door. She suggested to the public health nurse that, should she die, she would take the children with her. The children's father suffered from a mental illness, and had been violent and incarcerated in the past. While he was not living with the family, Ms S. was inconsistent regarding the contact he had with her and the children. The birth of Tara exacerbated Ms S.'s symptoms, and the children were placed in foster care, as they were felt to be at risk, given their mother's delusions and her increasingly detached attitude towards them. Ms S. remained in hospital for several months before being discharged on medication. She then obtained a disability pension and a two-bedroom apartment. She attended weekly supervised visits at the child welfare offices; over time, she demonstrated poor compliance with psychiatric follow-up.

During the assessment, it became clear that Tony and, in particular, Jane had a strong attachment to their mother as well as to each other. Tara had been in foster care since birth and demonstrated only a familiarity with her mother and siblings. Ms S.'s extended family minimized the degree to which she experienced delusions and appeared unable to offer her emotional support or financial resources. As a parent, Ms S. had functioned at least adequately for five years; during this time, community reports made limited or no mention of paranoid symptoms, indicating that her illness was in the developing stages. In hospital, her diagnosis remained puzzling; however, it was clear that her disorder was of a paranoid nature, possibly schizophrenia. Since being discharged from hospital, Ms S. had been able to care for herself, despite the fact that she continued to suffer from paranoid delusions. She remained suspicious of professionals, and lacked insight into the effect of her behaviour on the children.

During the supervised visits, it was observed that Jane had been deeply affected by the loss of her mother, as well as the inconsistencies of her mother's parenting. She presented as insecure and anxious about her family and displayed a negative self-image. When stressed, she exhibited maladaptive coping skills, such as withdrawing from those around her, destroying her own or other's possessions, or socializing with peers who got into trouble. A more positive characteristic was Jane's ability to recognize that her mother had serious problems which were not her fault. Tony appeared more happy than his sister, but tended to be more verbally inhibited. When asked about his mother and family, he appeared confused and unsure of his answers. Both children appeared comfortable living in their foster home.

Ms S. alternated between treating Jane affectionately and being extremely critical of her. She related to Tony in a more neutral fashion. Her interest in all the children varied from being attentive to vacant and unresponsive. Without improvement in areas of Ms S.'s parenting skills and increased emotional involvement, it was felt that the children would be at risk if left in her care. Ms S.'s style of isolating herself from family and professionals also remained a serious concern. Should the children return to her, it would have become difficult to maintain contact and monitor their safety.

Intervention

The assessor arranged a series of parent–children sessions in order to work with the family. It was recognized that the court assessor could be perceived as intimidating by the parent, which might impede the therapeutic process. In this case, however, the alternative was to introduce another person to a paranoid client, who was already feeling overwhelmed and suspicious of the many professionals with whom she had to work. Since a positive connection had been established between the clinician and client, it was felt that another therapist would only further confound the situation. The goal of the joint sessions was to assist Ms S. in making the visits a more interactive and positive experience for the children, whose positive response would then reward the mother.

In the initial sessions, the clinician intervened minimally in order to observe Ms S.'s style of interacting with her children. In subsequent individual sessions, the clinician offered simple, supportive suggestions regarding ways the mother could respond to the children (i.e., more verbal comments of praise). Ms S. made initial gains, and it became clear that, on a one-to-one basis, she was able to handle the demands of each child. If approached slowly and gently by the clinician, she was able to follow-through with suggestions to which the children, Jane in particular, responded positively.

Over time, however, Ms S.'s psychiatric symptoms began to overwhelm her and, increasingly, the delusions distracted her from appropriately focusing on the children. At times she would share bizarre thoughts with the older children, who appeared confused by their mother's behaviour. Ms S. terminated contact with the hospital and refused medical intervention or medication to control her delusions. As her psychiatric condition deteriorated and she became more isolated, the clinicians felt that persisting with the sessions would be too stressful for both her and the children. A concern then arose regarding the prolonged impact on the children of their mother's style of behaviour; she alternated from interest and affection, to indifference and criticism. The clinicians considered whether this experience would be more detrimental than the partial or total loss of the maternal relationship. There was also a renewed concern that Ms S. would incorporate the children into her delusional system, and this might compromise their physical safety. Despite her inconsistent behaviour and emotional presentation within the sessions, she was able to attend the visits regularly.

Outcome
The application of the Parenting Capacity guidelines enabled the assessors to clarify those areas of parenting which were of serious concern. Ms S. displayed several problem behaviours which affected her judgment regarding the children (guidelines 4 and 7). She alternated among affection, criticism, and lack of interest in the children. She incorporated the children into her paranoid delusions and then shared these thoughts. Ms S. became unable to relate to and maintain productive, consistent relationships with the professional supports (guidelines 8 and 9) which were available to her (i.e., the Children's Aid Society worker, Family Court Clinic assessor, psychiatrist) and tended to isolate herself from her family and friends. If placed with their mother, the children would clearly be at risk. Ms S. also had difficulty accepting responsibility for the concerns raised about her somewhat secretive relationship with the children's father, who had a history of extreme violence. Throughout the assessment she was inconsistent when she described this relationship. Furthermore, she was unable to recognize the impact of her disorder on her behaviour and judgment. Over time, she repeatedly denied that she suffered from any type of illness (guideline 6).

It became clear to the assessors that the children could not return to the custody of their mother. Given Tara's lack of attachment to her mother and sisters, it was recommended, and accepted by the court, that her needs would best be served by adoption rather than long-term foster care. A dilemma arose when the clinicians had to decide whether to continue visits between the older children and their mother, given that, at times, these were not a positive experience. The assessment had revealed a strong connection between Jane and her mother; both children had memories and experiences of a caring, attentive parent. While terminating access would allow them to settle in their long-term placement, it would deny the reality of their attachment to their natural parent. Consequently, it was recommended that the older children continue to have supervised visitation with their mother, who was again referred for psychiatric treatment. Despite Ms S.'s impairment, she was able to recognize that lack of follow-through could lead to the complete loss of her children. The clinicians hoped that the recommendations would motivate her to follow-through with treatment. Approximately one year after the assessment, Ms S. made contact with the psychiatrist. In the interim, she had consistently attended the supervised visits, and the children had remained in the same foster home. While she remained unable to resume parenting them, the visitation prevented the children from feeling they had been abandoned, and allowed Ms S. to maintain a minimal connection with the children's lives. In this case, with the coordinated efforts of the foster parent and the child welfare workers, the children were able to tolerate the feelings generated by these visits, and problem behaviours were not observed.

*Discussion*

As is illustrated by the case of Ms S., assessing parenting capacity usually occurs when there is a clinical concern regarding marginally or poorly functioning parents. In many cases, appropriate clinical interventions assist the parents in acquiring the skills necessary to prevent the dissolution of the family. In those situations where this is not successful, a clinician must carefully consider the decision to suspend temporarily or end parental rights. Termination of parental rights is an emotional and controversial topic in both clinical practice and family law. Given the unfortunate reality of breakdown in foster and group-home placements, as well as in adoptions, the decision to permanently remove a child is often fraught with conflict. These dilemmas include the rights of the parents to adequate time for improvement versus those of the child to a stable home; the influence of partners; assessing parent's ability to utilize community supports within the realities of the child welfare system; and, finally, the issue of visitation.

The last decade has seen a great interest in ensuring that individual's rights are protected by law. In situations where parents are moderately or severely debilitated by mental illness, the rights of the child may conflict with the rights of the parents. Parents are entitled to the opportunity to improve their skills or situation, yet a child also has the right to the opportunity for growth in a healthy, nurturing environment. Clinicians must struggle with the question of how long one should wait for a parent to demonstrate gains before making the decision to remove a child permanently. Inherent in this dilemma is the wish to preserve, as much as possible, the parenting, attachment, and family life that occurred prior to the parent's deterioration. This must be done without subjecting the child to damaging, long-term uncertainty about his or her primary caregivers and residence. With a psychiatric impairment, the parent's rate of improvement may be very slow as a result of such factors as social and economic circumstances, and the nature of the illness itself. Particularly in the case of a very young child or infant, such as Tara, immediate permanency planning is of paramount importance if further damage to development is to be prevented.

In these situations, the clinician should wait until it has been determined whether the recovery of the parent can be expected within a time frame that will safeguard the development of the child. This requires a thorough psychiatric examination and a psychosocial evaluation, as has been described in the Parenting Capacity guidelines.

When considering the client's social functioning and social supports, the clinician must carefully evaluate the influence of partners or spouses. A partner may exercise enormous influence on a parent's coping ability, and on his or her general disposition towards parenting. When a partner is able to stabilize and support the home situation, his or her presence can be reassuring and supportive for the children. In some cases, this individual may eventually become the primary attachment figure and a crucial support person who can sustain the viability of the family. In other situations, however, the partner may severely exacerbate problems. This can be particularly difficult in cases where both partners suffer from a mental illness or personality disorder which affects their ability to establish organized routines and exercise good parental judgment. At times, a parent who demonstrates some basic skills may be unable to recognize that he or she is being undermined, negatively influenced, or abused by a partner, thus placing the children at risk. Often, considerable professional time is spent trying to convince the parent to leave his or her spouse in order to ensure that the children are protected. In situations where this is unsuccessful, the parent is unable to place the interests of the children above those of the adults. With support, however, it is possible that the natural parent will deal with the problematic relationship, and the family can remain intact.

Assessing parents' ability to form a therapeutic alliance and utilize community supports may also become a serious dilemma. Often, the more dysfunctional families with a mentally ill parent have attended multiple community services, and have not followed-through with recommended treatment. They are seen as being unable to engage in a therapeutic alliance. This may be true of those parents who are influenced by a transient and chaotic lifestyle, and exhibit a pattern of repeatedly attributing lack of follow-through to external or situational factors, such as lack of finances or inconveniently scheduled appointments.

In other cases, however, lack of follow-through can be attributed to the high rate of staff turnover in the child welfare and children's mental health settings. While this factor is often dismissed as insignificant, it does contribute to clients' inability to form a therapeutic alliance. Given their own negative childhood experiences and the problems associated with mental illness, a large number of disadvantaged parents experience difficulties establishing and maintaining interpersonal relationships. They are also unable to manage multiple relationships with professionals simultaneously. Ironically, in an attempt to provide comprehensive service, plans of care or intervention often require parents to engage simultaneously with several helping professionals. A lack of coordination and clear role definition between these agencies or individuals may undermine any gains the parent might be able to make. It is interesting to note that the more chaotic families often have a equally chaotic history of multiple workers and underuse of services. In some instances, it may be more useful to reduce the number of professionals involved and assign one or two intensive helpers to the parent. Coordination among the professionals, such as the lawyer, psychiatrist, and social worker, ensures a more effective plan as it is more productive to work with these complex and multiproblem families with a collaborative rather than adversarial approach. For example, while Ms S. waited sixteen months to become involved with a psychiatrist, her lawyer did play a pivotal role in encouraging her to attend. Rather than simply offering verbal encouragement, Ms S.'s counsel monitored involvement with the psychiatrist and was interested in Ms S.'s recovery.

In cases where professional help has not been consistent and collaborative, and the child has been in care for an extended period of time, a new dilemma arises. An important question to consider is whether the system provided the parent with the appropriate resources to make gains or whether the system, by its very nature, impeded the parent's progress. In these cases, it is very difficult to determine whether the child's interests would be served by continuing to remain in foster care in order to give the natural parent a well-planned opportunity to improve, or by being permanently separated from the parent, given the length of time he or she has already been in care. In situations where the child has and will continue to receive stable, consistent foster care, and the parent exhibits positive signs for recovery (such as an interest in the child and an ability to work with support systems), it may be in the child's interest to allow the parent more time. In those instances where the child has endured multiple foster placements or has special developmental needs, and the parent's prognosis is marginal or poor, it would not be in the child's interests to delay permanency planning.

When parental illness and circumstances are so severe that there will be an inevitable dissolution of the family, the age of the child is an important consideration during permanency planning. Perhaps some of the most difficult and complex decisions involve the older child who has developed an attachment to the ill parent with whom the child has resided for several years. Once custodial matters have been determined, the question of access must be considered. Access may be contraindicated in cases of severe neglect or abuse, and where there is a strong negative association with the absent parent. However, in other situations, as with Ms S., Jane, and Tony, visits could serve to preserve some aspects of the relationship with the primary attachment figure, and prevent the children from feeling rejected or abandoned. In the case example, Jane, who worried about her mother's well-being, was reassured by seeing her mother during the visits.

Decisions surrounding visitation should address three areas: (1) the historical nature of the parent–child relationship, and whether the child has positive memories or extremely negative associations with his or her parent; (2) the age, temperament, and developmental level of the child, as some older or more resilient children may tolerate well the stress of visitation, while younger more vulnerable children may become very unsettled by repeated exposure to the parent; and (3) the wishes of the child. The dilemma in these situations is that a successful visitation experience for the child requires a therapeutic component, which unfortunately is not incorporated into the process. Parents may need support and education about how to approach their children, while children require assistance in working out the complex feelings generated by the visits. Often the child's response is handled by a foster parent who observes an upset or irritable child return home from a visit. The foster parent is unsure what provoked this reaction, and may mistakenly attribute it simply to see-ing the absent parent. A combination of therapy and visitation greatly assists the child in mourning the loss of the parent. A failure to provide this can encourage a child to maintain the hope for family reunification in situations where this is not possible. It is very important that children appropriately process their feelings and receive education and reassur-ance that the parent's illness is not their fault. Unfortunately, a lack of resources prevents child welfare and children's mental health settings from offering therapeutic visitation services. While this area has been rel-atively unexplored in the literature, it is of increasing interest to clini-cians in the mental health field.

## Conclusion

The enormous implications of these types of decisions point to the need for clinicians in the child welfare field to have specialized training in assessing parenting capacity and planning for families where one or both parents suffer from a mental illness. Research in the field has shown that children of the mentally ill are at increased risk for problems in their adjustment. However, there are protective factors which, if present, allow a child to remain with a disturbed parent and have minimal difficulties in adulthood. The Toronto Parenting Capacity Assessment Project has attempted to provide a standardized set of criteria which should be used when determining a parent's capacity to care for a child. In those instances where mental illness prevents a parent from assuming full-time responsibility for a child, the advisability of visitation must be carefully considered. This essay has presented the theoretical and research mate-rial which has contributed to the field. The Parenting Capacity guidelines assist in this decision-making process, as was illustrated by the case of Ms S. and her children. Finally, the authors have outlined a number of dilemmas which are regularly encountered when working with these fam-ilies. As the theoretical, clinical, and research literature develops, it is hoped that more effective and innovative interventions for both parents and children will be developed within the child welfare and children's mental health fields.

REFERENCES

Barnum, R. (1987). Clinical experience – understanding controversies in visita-tion. *Journal of American Academy of Child and Adolescent Psychiatry, 26,* 788–792.

Cicchetti, D. (1987, May). The developmental psychopathology of the affective disorders. Paper presented at the meeting of the Society for Research in Child Development, Baltimore, MD.

Dodge, K. (1990). Developmental psychopathology in children of depressed mothers. *Developmental Psychology, 26* (1), 3–6.

Gelfand, D., & Teti, D. (1990). The effects of maternal depression on children. *Clinical Psychology Review, 10,* 329–353.

Goodman S., & Brumley, E. (1990). Schizophrenic and depressed mothers: Relational deficits in parenting. *Developmental Psychology, 26,* 31–39.

Hafner, J. (1986). *Marriage and mental illness.* New York: Guilford.

Keller, M., Beardslee, W., Dorer, D., Lavori, P., Samuelson, H., & Klerman, G. (1986). Impact of severity and chronicity of parental affective illness on adaptive functioning and psychopathology in children. *Archives of General Psychiatry, 43,* 930–937.

Laroche, C., Sheiner, R., Lester, E., Benierakis, C., Marrache, M., Engelsmann, F., & Cheifetz, P. (1987). Children of parents with manic depressive illness: A follow-up study. *Canadian Journal of Psychiatry, 32,* 563–569.

Patterson, G.R. (1982). *A social learning approach: Coercive family processes.* Eugene, OR: Castalia.

Rosenthal, D. (1970). *Genetic theory and abnormal behavior.* New York: McGraw-Hill.

Rubin, K.H. (1987, April). Predicting childhood depression. Paper presented at the meeting of the Society for Research in Child Development, Baltimore, MD.

Rutter, M. (1990). Commentary: Some focus and process considerations regarding effects of parental depression on children. *Developmental Psychology, 26* (1), 60–67.

Sameroff, A., Barocas, R., & Seifer, R. (1984). The early development of children born to mentally ill women. In N. Watt, J. Anthony, L. Wynne, & J. Rolf (Eds.), *Children at risk for schizophrenia* (pp. 482–514). New York: Cambridge University Press.

Seifer, R., & Sameroff, A. (1981). Adaptive behaviour in young children of emotionally disturbed women. *Journal of Applied Developmental Psychology, 1,* 251–276.

Steinhauer, P. (1991). *The least detrimental alternative: A systemic guide to case planning and decision making for children in care.* Toronto: University of Toronto Press.

Walker, E., Downey, G., & Bergman, A. (1989). The effects of parental psychopathology and maltreatment on child behaviour: A test of the diathesis-stress model. *Child Development, 60,* 15–24.

Weintraub, S. (1987). Risk factors in schizophrenia: The Stony Brook high-risk project. *Schizophrenia Bulletin, 13,* 439–449.

Weissman, M.M., & Boyd, J.H. (1985). Affective disorders: Epidemiology. In H.I. Kaplan, A.M. Freedman, & B.J. Sadock (Eds.), *Comprehensive textbook of psychiatry* (4th ed.) (pp. 764–769). Baltimore, MD: Williams & Wilkins.

Werner, E., & Smith, R. (1982). *Vulnerable but invincible.* New York: McGraw-Hill.

# Loss of Parents through Mental Illness: The Recovery of a Six-Year-Old Boy

DEBRA MacRAE

When parental mental illness impairs the ability to provide adequate basic care for a child, and when the support of family members or community services cannot remedy this situation, it is necessary for parental custodial rights to be terminated. Though many mentally ill parents can provide adequate care for their children, others cannot. This essay discusses the unfortunate circumstances in which parental mental illness causes children to be permanently separated from their parents and describes the treatment of one young boy who has suffered this loss. Many of the presenting features of this case are typical of child welfare referrals assessed at the Family Court Clinic of the Clarke Institute of Psychiatry, in Toronto, Ontario. These children commonly have had to cope with chronic strain or trauma for an extended time during early development. Consequently, psychological development is impaired. It appears that, with the provision of 'good enough' substitute parents, and appropriate treatment, it is possible for some of these children to overcome their psychological delays and attain healthy functioning.

Following a general overview of the issues, case material is presented from a developmental perspective. Theoretical discussions are interspersed within the material. Various psychoanalytic models have been used to explain the child's behaviour and development. The application of multiple theoretical models to the understanding of clinical material has been advocated by Fred Pine (1990). The author of this paper is in agreement with Dr Pine's multi-model perspective. The essay concludes with a discussion of how therapy can assist children who have lost their parents through mental illness.

In the Court Clinic, the primary issue to be assessed is the effect of mental illness on parenting ability. Where the parenting deficits are so severe as to jeopardize the safety or healthy development of the child, and when there is little or no hope for improvement by the parent, the clinic subscribes to the view that it is necessary to provide alternative care for the child (Goldstein, Freud, & Solnit, 1973; 1979).

In today's social and legal climate, much emphasis is placed on maintaining the integrity of the family unit. In practice, this means attempting to ameliorate family dysfunction through the provision of community services. Where such an approach is successful, the benefits to the child are immeasurable. However, in a number of instances, this approach has proven unsuccessful. Consequently, much of the young life of the child has been characterized by chronic abuse and/or neglect. Cumulatively, these problems constitute a degree of risk that warrants an apprehension. Very often, these concerns climax with a specific event that results in an immediate apprehension. Such an event may represent a significant trauma for the child. However, it is crucial that the significance of chronic neglect or abuse not be overlooked.

In cases where the legal tie between the parent and child must be severed, there have been extreme failures in the caregiving environment (Goldstein, Freud, & Solnit, 1973; 1979). Within the referral population of the Family Court Clinic, many of the parents have been diagnosed with either a major psychiatric illness or a character disorder, or both. While these may cause family problems at one level (i.e., psychosis, psychological withdrawal, aggression, etc.), other factors also contribute significantly to family dysfunction. In exploring the personal history of the parents, one often finds evidence that their style of parenting echoes conscious and unconscious memories of their own experiences in childhood.

The role of genetic heritability in psychiatric illness is not yet fully understood, though it is generally accepted that illness in the parent increases the risk for the child (Rutter & Quinton, 1984; Emde, 1988; Seifer & Samaroff, 1981; Samaroff, Barochas, & Seifer, 1984; Weintraub, 1987; Anthony, 1983; Main & Goldwyn, 1984). Authors such as Rutter and Quinton (1984) and Emde (1988) acknowledge genetic heritability, but have emphasized the role of the environment in contributing to psychiatric disorders in childhood. Emde (1988), in particular, emphasized the 'specificity of the environment,' distinguishing one child's experience within a family from that of a sibling raised in the same environment.

The loss of a parent through mental illness is an underdeveloped subject in the literature. This in itself reflects the paradoxical nature of the issue in that permanent separation from parents is likely to be subsumed under other topics such as child maltreatment, fostering, or adoption.

The literature on the loss of a parent through death, divorce, or adoption is valuable in that it delineates the process of mourning and highlights important details pertaining to such factors as gender, relational issues, and developmental phases (Furman, 1974, 1986; Raphael, 1983; Nickman, 1985; Rutter, 1971; Cohen, 1990). These are also significant in the loss of a parent through mental illness. Erna Furman (1974, p. 47) contends that bereavement is more complex and prolonged where there is no actual death. She argues further that the death of a parent is not necessarily traumatic: 'different combinations of internal and external factors proved to have been traumatogenic' (pp. 192–193). In working with children who have lost their parents through mental illness, it becomes clear that often separation from the parent is but one painful event in what has been a generally traumatized young life.

For the children seen at the Family Court Clinic, other factors such as chronic neglect and/or physical or sexual abuse are also a part of their traumatic history. Given that the trauma has often been inflicted on the child by the parent, the subsequent loss of that parent is likely to be experienced differently from the loss of a parent through death or divorce. The chronicity of severe parent–child problems may constitute the most significant trauma for the child. If this is the case, the actual loss of the parent is secondary to the primary trauma of chronic neglect and abuse.

With regard to the child's emotional response to the loss of the parent, it is very difficult for mourning to take place. Freud described melancholia as occurring when there has been significant disappointment in the relationship with the lost object. Where such disappointment exists, there is a strong identification with the lost object with the result of 'an extraordinary diminution in self regard' (Freud, 1917). Freud further stated that, where such an identification takes place, 'the love relation need not be given up' (1917, p. 249). It is easier to give up the real relationship with the good object when it has been internalized as nurturing and reasonably satisfying. Where this does not occur, there is a tenacious effort to cling to the real relationship in the hope of getting basic needs met. The child believes that he was bad, in contrast to his parents, and that his innate badness caused the family breakdown. Since a good-enough object has not yet been internalized, the child has no other recourse than to idealize the parent and denigrate the self. This can change with therapy, in proportion with the improvement of internalized self and object representations. That is, the resolution of mourning can occur once a sense of good-enough objects (parental figures) and a sense of a good-enough self have been established.

According to object-relations theory, any child who has spent a significant amount of time with any parent will have a psychological relationship with that parent that will endure beyond even permanent separation. (See Greenberg and Mitchell [1983] for an overview of the major object-relations theorists.) Accordingly, conscious and unconscious memories and representations survive such a separation. Factors such as the age of the child at the time of the separation, the amount of time spent in the care of the natural parent, the degree of trauma experienced while in the care of the parent, and the innate constitution of the child colour and shape a child's personality and have a profound influence on his or her sense of self (Freud, 1917; Kohut, 1977). When self and object (other) representations become structured by traumatic experiences, future functioning and relationships are also affected, or determined, by these experiences (Freud, 1917).

It is critical that the child's experience amidst the chaos and confusion of family breakdown be understood so that the suffering of the child can be relieved and healthy psychological development can be promoted. Farber and Egeland (1987) p. 254 have emphasized that 'there is no consistent or typical personality profile of abused children. It is not surprising that there is no predictable pattern of maladaptation, considering that the abusive situation and "abusive environment" are highly varied from one case to another.' Though each child will be affected in a unique way, the maltreatment literature has consistently shown that these children suffer developmental delays that cause them to be disturbed in many areas of their functioning (Aber & Cicchetti, 1984), including the lack of opportunity to develop sufficient psychological structures, such as a sense of safety and security, positive self-esteem, positive expectations of relations with others, and a reliable ability to control strong impulses and behave in socially adaptive ways.

Psychotherapy with a six-year-old boy who had lost his parents through mental illness revealed how his psychological development had been impaired by the deprivation and abuse he had suffered in his early years. This discussion describes his recovery through the provision of an adequate caregiving environment and intensive psychotherapy. Therapy was geared towards understanding the impact of the traumatic experiences on the child, and using this to repair and mobilize psychological growth.

*Case History*

Alex was referred for psychotherapy at age five years, ten months. He had

depressive symptoms such as inhibition, fragile self-esteem, and somatiza-
tion (headaches and stomach aches with no apparent physical cause). He
was described as a frightened, nervous little boy who worried that adults
would abandon him. He was also excessively clingy and terrified of strang-
ers. He longed to be best at everything, and became unhappy and sullen
when he failed to achieve this ideal. He was seen as sensitive and caring in
relation to family members; however, he had difficulty managing his
anger and occasionally threatened adults with a hockey stick.

Despite his above-average intelligence, Alex's academic performance
was in the low to middle range. He had strengths in verbal expression,
but his fine motor coordination and ability to draw were particularly
poor. He was described as a loner, with no special friends, who occasionally physically attacked other children.

Alex was the first-born child of a nineteen-year-old woman who was
diagnosed with depression. His father was a twenty-year-old man who suffered from alcoholism and an apparent borderline personality disorder.
Alex's early development was described as normal, though he always slept
with his mother, was a bed-wetter, and was anxious in the presence of his
father. He frequently witnessed his father beating his mother, and when
he was one and a half years old, his father began to scream at him and
slap his face. When he was three, Alex's mother abandoned him to his
abusive father. Alex was undernourished and unkempt in the care of his
father. When Alex was about three and a half years old, his father burned
his hands on a stove. Alex was apprehended and placed with his maternal
grandparents. After two and a half years of court proceedings, this placement was made permanent. Alex had supervised visits with his father and
unsupervised visits with his mother. The quality and frequency of his contact with his parents had been variable. The access appears to have prevented him from idealizing his parents. This probably has contributed to
his contentment in living with his grandparents.

Alex's move to his grandparent's home constituted the beginning of
growth-enhancing parent–child relations for this young boy. However, it
is evident in the details of the presenting complaints that Alex suffered
from poor self-esteem and a chronic expectation of neglectful or abusive
relations with others. From an object-relations perspective, this meant
that Alex's memories of bad experiences had accrued to form a series of
self and object representations that served to organize his perception of
his self and his world. These perceptions were unconscious for the most
part, and had become structured to the degree that new, more positive
experiences were ineffectual in bringing adequate relief to Alex's painful

inner world. He required intensive psychotherapy to help him internalize the new and essentially positive relations that he now experienced.

## The Treatment

In his paper 'Remembering, repeating and working through,' Freud (1914) described that aspect of a transference relationship wherein 'the patient does not remember anything of what he has forgotten and repressed, but acts it out. He reproduces it, not as a memory, but as an action; he repeats it, without, of course, knowing [that he is doing so]' (1914, p. 150). It was emphasized that 'the patient will begin his treatment with a repetition of this kind' (Freud, 1914, p. 150). This was true of Alex's therapy. He immediately developed a transference relationship in which he repeated themes of the abuse, deprivation, and abandonment. This behaviour was not a conscious recollection of these experiences, as is evident in the material wherein the memories are represented by symbolism. Rather, the behaviour was a re-enactment of experiences repressed from consciousness.

In addition to the working-through of painful memories, Alex used the transference to redress deficits in the development of his personality. This included a maternal transference, wherein he developed a sense of safety and security and sought out interactions that provided the narcissistic mirroring of which he had been deprived in his early years. This led to more positive self and object representations and to a shift into the phallic-narcissistic phase of development, where his self-esteem was further advanced and consolidated. Parallel to this work was a sado-masochistic transference, the resolution of which contributed to his learning impulse control and more appropriate ways of being close to others. Having consolidated the earlier psychological structures, as noted above, and advancing in his cognitive development, Alex was able to move to more age-appropriate functioning centring on a prelatency paternal transference. In this phase of treatment, Alex worked on issues of rivalry, competition, identification with the same gendered parent, and the surrendering of magical omnipotence to the recognition of external reality and rules. Subsequently he focused on latency forms of play, often looking to the therapist as a teacher–father figure. This period included a great emphasis on sharpening his cognitive skills.

The following case material demonstrates the advances in Alex's personality development as outlined above. As is necessary in the synopsis of any long-term treatment, the content and sequence of Alex's therapy are artificially simplified. Nevertheless, core issues are delineated to highlight some of the most salient aspects of the work.

Throughout the first few months of therapy, Alex focused on issues of safety and security. The beginning manifestations of this theme were represented in the early sessions, when Alex expressed his fear of danger and his need for protection. Alex would frequently stand on the inside window-ledge of the therapist's ninth-storey office and press against the window-pane. At these times, the therapist placed her arm firmly between Alex and the window, and spoke to him about how he felt that he was in danger and needed to feel held, to feel protected, and to feel safe. The same scene was played out in the stairwell, where Alex would recklessly hurtle over the banister, requiring the therapist to move in and catch him. Alex was caught on each occasion, and this behaviour was again explained to him as his concern regarding lack of safety and his wish to be protected. After many repetitions, this behaviour subsided, and Alex's journey down the stairwell became more typically achieved by sliding down the banister. This appeared to be fun, but still required the therapist's close attention and availability.

The maternal transference was elaborated within the beginning months of his treatment. An unconscious theme that Alex raised early in the therapy was his fear of abandonment. He was unable to talk about why he doesn't live with Mommy and scribbled on paper with a black marker. When the therapist stated that he was probably very angry at Mommy because of not living with her and noted that his drawing was very black, he said, 'No it's not!' and desperately tried to colour it blue. He responded positively to the therapist's ongoing empathy with his terrible sense of being left by the people that he needs and loves. Talking about his need to not be abandoned validated Alex's need to feel secure.

His perception of the relations between mothers and fathers and babies or small children were persistently bleak early in the therapy. This was apparent in the evolving transference, where themes of a neglected, abused, and greedy baby developed alongside themes of a fighting family, sibling rivalry, and an early and desperate need for narcissistic reflection. He played out battle scenes in the doll house, where all of the family figures were brutally killed. The father doll would beat the baby doll, and the baby would cry desperately for its mother to come and help. The mother would come, call it a 'sucky baby,' and kick it in the face. His emotional deprivation was evident in themes of hunger. He told a story of Jack and the Beanstock in which Jack tried to wake his mother up to go get the beans but had to go get them himself. His sense of deprivation led to recognition of the strength of his neediness, which frightened him considerably.

Increasingly, he expressed concerns about being greedy. He spoke of how his grandma spent lots of money on toys for him and how he wished that she would keep her money for food or for bingo. In his play, he also expressed the worry that his therapy was too costly for his grandparents. This concern about resources led to a discussion of how very needy Alex felt. This was extended to his worry that he would take too much and somehow hurt the people that he needs, and that then they would not be there for him any more.

The development of a basic sense of safety and security are among the earliest of the infant's psychological achievements. As Alex came to consolidate a sense of safety and security within the therapy, he began to develop play themes wherein he sought out early infantile mirroring interactions with the therapist. The play became organized in such a way that the therapist was mirroring Alex's movements and sounds. In this, Alex seemed like a little baby lying back on a blanket, waiting expectantly for Mother to communicate her interest in him by engaging him in play. Stern (1985) suggested that a mother's exciting play is a central motivating factor in the baby's efforts to organize perceptions and engage at an affective level with the world. The mother helps the baby discover its self and the self's range of possibilities for feeling states and modes of communication. This in turn 'regulates the feeling of attachment, physical proximity, and security' (Stern, 1985, p. 102). It seemed that these were the needs that Alex wanted the therapist to attend to. While this therapist might often persist in encouraging a child to elaborate upon his or her own themes, she accepted Alex's directive to perform for him at that particular time in his therapy. Though Alex appeared to enjoy this, he sometimes appeared to find it overstimulating and he lashed out furiously, throwing several toys at the therapist. His rage in relation to his lack of appropriate mirroring was clear. When the therapist contained this behaviour, Alex lay down on the floor like a baby and made a gesture as though raising a bottle to his mouth. However, in this case, the 'bottle' was the sharp end of a pair of scissors. He opened and closed the scissors in his mouth. Here, Alex's rage turned to helplessness, and then to depression, which led to masochistic behaviour. Accordingly, he turned his destructive impulses towards himself.

Running parallel to the themes of early infantile mirroring and phallic narcissism was a sado-masochistic transference that reflected the psychological damage that had accrued from his neglect and physical abuse. Alex's play and manner of relating to the therapist became increasingly sadistic. He played 'Doctor' with the therapist, and rather than providing care, he whacked her on the knees with a ruler to test her reflexes, or across the chest to check her heart rate. He gave the therapist medicine by symbolically shooting it down her throat with a gun. He threw things at her, beginning with a truck and the daddy doll. The therapist consistently redirected this activity to his play with the dolls, and Alex laughed sadistically when the therapist made sounds of victims whimpering in pain. Although this behaviour was repeatedly contained and redirected by the therapist, it persisted for some time. Alex continually created new, seemingly innocent games that would escalate into aggression against the therapist or masochistic behaviour against himself.

Novick and Novick (1991) linked sado-masochistic character pathology with a delusion of omnipotence. They suggested that this omnipotence resulted from the child's experience, when 'as infants, their inborn capacities to elicit needed responses were often ineffectual. Their mothers were depressed or anxious and only smiled when they emerged from these states, not in response to the child's smile ... They associate their mothers with pain' (p. 216). They also described how masochism creates 'a sense of suffering reunion with the object' (p. 217) and concluded that these 'children fell back on omnipotent fantasies of control to maintain their self-esteem' (p. 17). Ornstein (1991) rejected the idea of sadism as the product of an aggressive drive and substituted this classical perspective with the notion that sadism is 'the expression of chronic narcissistic rage, which arises in relation to narcissistic vulnerability' (p. 222). She linked sadistic behaviour with trauma, where 'the developmentally needed self/object responsiveness was missing, [and] the patient as a child may have been actively mistreated and abused – situations where the child's emotional environment was unpredictable, volatile, and violent' (p. 223). Alex was an abused child, and his sado-masochistic behaviour was no doubt linked to that abuse. His search for mirroring in the transference suggested that he did not experience adequate positive interaction in his infancy. The narcissistic pain from this deprivation would be extreme, and would probably be linked to his proximity to his depressed mother. Thus, in the therapy, Alex's masochistic behaviour reflected a remembered way of being close to the maternal object. Alex's omnipotence in this behaviour served as a defence against narcissistic pain, and provided an illusory compensation for his poor self-esteem.

Alex's abusive and masochistic behaviour was contained by the therapist's directive to cease the play when the sado-masochism had become activated. This included making comments to Alex about how he seemed to think that this was a way of being close to other people, and references to his anger about not having felt safe when he was little. These sequences required many repetitions, and it was not until much later in the treatment, when he developed an idealizing paternal transference, that he was able to internalize the therapist's rules and incorporate them as a function of his own superego prohibitions.

As described below, there was a shift in the themes of Alex's play, and his manner of relating to the therapist. Alex had clearly made significant gains in developing more positive representations of self and object, and the relations between the two. Having achieved this, he was able to move forward in his development. The subsequent use of the transference indicated that Alex had shifted to phase dominance at the phallic-narcissistic level.

Edgcumbe and Burgner (1975) focused on the 'development of relationships to self and objects' (p. 163) during the phallic-narcissistic phase. They described the child's innate need for high levels of admiration from the object (the parents or their substitutes), and the need for positive identification with the same-sex parent. Given his dramatic early history, it is not surprising that Alex had not mastered the tasks of the phallic-narcissistic phase. However, with the critical changes in his external world (i.e., the move to his grandparents') and his gains in therapy, Alex moved rapidly from infantile ways of relating to himself and his object world to energetically engaging the challenges of the phallic-narcissistic phase.

With a small ball of play dough he initiated exciting games of hockey, golfing, snooker, and tennis. He exhibited his skill and daring for the therapist's admiration. With the same ball, he discovered a fact that the therapist had never suspected: her very small office could accommodate an entire baseball field. Increasingly, Alex was able to say, 'Hey – I'm good at this!' in an emphatic but somewhat surprised tone. The therapist agreed with him, saying 'Yes you are!' Alex then became Mad Max, a world pro golfer, and assigned the therapist the role of 'Debra the Star,' his major competitor, whom he always defeated. In this play, we see the beginnings of a more appropriate sublimation of his energies into activities that are creative and rewarding for Alex. We can also see the strengthening of his representation of a valued self, as he increasingly internalized the admiration provided in therapy.

One of the more complicated aspects of Alex's journey through the phallic-narcissistic phase was his need to identify with his father, who was a dangerously abusive man. Alex demonstrated this conflict in his play and was eventually able to speak of his fear that he too would be an abusive parent when he grew up. Alex longed for a father figure with whom to relate to and to identify. He woefully lamented the fact that the therapist was a woman. He passionately longed for rough play with a man. Mother's most recent partner was able to play a pivotal role in resolving this difficulty for Alex, as he proved to be a playful man who appreciated Alex's need for a father figure.

As Alex further consolidated his sense of self-esteem, there were increasing shifts in his object world, as was demonstrated in the therapy. In contrast to the earlier, sadistic doctor, a doctor came into the play who revived the injured and dead soldiers. Early in the therapy all of the family dolls were brutally killed in family battles. Increasingly, the boy doll was privileged with surviving the destruction. Finally, the baby doll was substituted for the boy doll as the sole survivor of the family battles. Alex allowed the therapist's assertion that there is something very special about the baby. When the family had all been killed off and the therapist asked, 'Who will care for the baby?,' the mother was tenderly revived and the baby was placed in her care.

Alex eventually busied himself with drawing self-representations with the message 'I love you' down the margin. He added various family names, including his 'mommy,' to the various drawings. The therapist supported his expression of love for all of the people in his family by telling him that his drawings were very beautiful.

From an object-relations perspective, Alex had now internalized the good-enough object. When his mother proposed to have him live with her, he suggested that this might be attractive in another five years. He no longer clung to an image of an idealized mother, but rather was able to appraise her in a more realistic manner. He was no longer identified with an abandoning object, nor was his self-esteem determined by this former identification. Though he valued visiting with his mother, he could confront her with how she disappointed him rather than blame himself. This was also true of his relationship with his father.

After one and a half years of treatment, Alex had consolidated sufficient psychological structure to advance to a prelatency level of psychological functioning. He became more interested in competing with the therapist, and Oedipal issues surfaced, with curiosity about adults sleeping together and some rivalry around fantasied boyfriends of the therapist, whom he imagined were listed in her 'black book of all the guys you dumped before you picked the final one.' He selected the head of the clinic as his Oedipal rival and contemptuously asked: 'Why is he called Dr Hood? Does he wear a hood all the time?' Kohut (1977) wrote that the Oedipal conflict is not particularly traumatic for the child when earlier psychological structure has been sufficiently consolidated. This appeared to be true for Alex, who was more preoccupied with a positive paternal transference than with competition for the maternal object. Alex idealized the therapist as a father figure, dreamily telling her that he loved her 'magical bunts' (in the baseball games). He requested lessons in bunting. Increasingly he could play by the rules, tolerate losing, and say that he could now play 'just for fun.' He also acknowledged his conflict about growing up. He enjoyed the sophistication of playing by real rules, but missed the fantasy of being able to win whenever he wanted to.

Alex's treatment is still in progress, and recently he has been increasingly engaging in appropriate latency levels of play. The energetic motor activity of his perpetual baseball games is gradually giving way to matters focused on concentration and thinking. He devotes more and more time to strategizing trades between major-league baseball players in an endeavour to outsmart the therapist. He is more and more attracted to board games, a particularly popular form of latency-age play. His school performance has improved dramatically and he is now able to play with other children without physically attacking them. When he has consolidated this latency-age level of functioning, the termination of therapy will commence.

Alex will never be entirely free from the pain of the memories of his early childhood. However, a change in environment and intensive psychotherapy have enabled him to move forward in his development and put more distance between him and these painful feelings. His inner world has changed immensely and now appears to be a far more habitable place.

*Discussion*

From the material that Alex brought to his therapy, it was clear that this child's self and object representations had become structured by the traumatic experiences of his early life. Despite the two years of improved environmental circumstances with his grandparents, Alex continued to feel worthless and expected to be abused and rejected. These were the repressed memories that he 'acted out' in the transference, and in his behaviour at school and at home. In the transference relationship, Alex repeated these experiences with the therapist as his mother, father, and self. In this context, and with many repetitions, Alex accrued more positive memories about interacting with parental figures. The transference also permitted Alex's demonstration of areas of need in terms of phase-appropriate responses from the parental object. This included early mirroring, toddler-age narcissistic reflection, and safe competition with a father substitute that eventually provided a positive identification figure for Alex.

These gains were hard won by Alex and the therapist. The counter-transference was particularly challenging throughout the sado-masochistic phase of the therapy, and the therapist sometimes experienced feelings of helplessness, rage, and an occasional wish to shake Alex and demand that he cease his abusive behaviour. Good supervision for the beginning therapist, or peer consultation for the more experienced therapist, can be critical in containing the intense feelings that such a transference engenders.

Many of the children seen at the Family Court Clinic have experienced deprivation or abuse, as Alex did in his early years. Removal from their family of origin is the first step in their recovery from chronic trauma. Therapy appears to contribute to the development of positive self and object representations so critical to healthy psychological functioning. Transference-based psychotherapy also allows the mastering of delayed areas of development. With careful placement planning, and appropriate psychotherapy, the loss of a parent through mental illness can become a sad but tolerable part of a child's history, rather than a lifelong tragedy.

REFERENCES

Aber, J., & Cicchetti, D. (1984). The socio-emotional development of maltreated children: An empirical and theoretical analysis. In H. Fitzgerald, B. Lester, & M. Yogman (Eds.), *Theory and research in behavioral paediatrics, Vol. II* (pp. 147–205). New York: Plenum.

Anthony, E.J. (1983). Infancy in a crazy environment In J.D. Call, E. Galenson, & R.L. Tyson (Eds.), *Frontiers of infant psychiatry* (pp. 95–114). New York: Basic Books.

Blos, P., Jr. (1991). Sadomasochism and the defense against recall of painful affect. *Journal of the American Psychoanalytic Association, 39*, 417–430.

Blum, H.P. (1991). Sadomasochism in the psychoanalytic process, within and beyond the pleasure principle: Discussion. *Journal of the American Psychoanalytic Association, 39*, 431–450.

Cicchetti, D. (1987). Developmental psychopathology in infancy: Illustration from the study of maltreated youngsters. *Journal of Consulting and Clinical Psychology, 55*, 837–845.

Chused, J.F. (1988). The transference neurosis in child analysis. *The Psychoanalytic Study of the Child, 43*, 51–81.

Cohen, D.J. (1990). Enduring sadness: Early loss, vulnerability, and the shaping of character. *The Psychoanalytic Study of the Child, 45*, 157–177.

Edgcumbe, R., & Burgner, M. (1975). The phallic-narcissistic phase: A differentiation between preoedipal and oedipal aspects of phallic development. *The Psychoanalytic Study of the Child, 3*, 161–180.

Emde, R.N. (1988). Development terminable and interminable: Innate and motivational factors from infancy. *International Journal of Psychoanalysis, 69*, 23–42.

Farber, E.A., & Egeland, B. (1987). Invulnerability among abused and neglected children. In E.J. Anthony & B.J. Cohler (Eds.), *The invulnerable child* (pp. 253–288). New York: Guilford.

Freud, S. (1917). Mourning and melancholia. *SE, 14*, 243–257.

Freud, S. (1914). Remembering, repeating and working-through. *SE, 12*, 147–156.

Furman, E. (1974). *A child's parent dies: Studies in childhood bereavement.* London: Yale University Press.

Furman, E. (1986). On trauma: When is the death of a parent traumatic. *The Psychoanalytic Study of the Child, 41*, 191–208.

Goldstein, J., Freud, A., & Solnit, A. (1973). *Beyond the best interests of the child.* New York: Free Press.

Goldstein, J., Freud, A., & Solnit, A. (1979). *Before the best interests of the child.* New York: Free Press.

Greenberg, J.R., & Mitchell, S.A. (1983). *Object relations in psychoanalytic theory.* London: Harvard University Press.

Kernberg, O.F. (1991). Sadomasochism, sexual excitement and perversion. *Journal of the American Psychoanalytic Association, 39*, 333–361.

Kohut, H. (1977). *The restoration of the self.* New York: International Universities Press.

Khan, M.M., & Masud, R. (1963). The concept of cumulative trauma. *The Psychoanalytic Study of the Child, 18*, 286–306.

Main, M., & Goldwyn, R. (1984). Predicting rejection of her infant from mother's representation of her own experience: Implications for the abused-abusing intergenerational cycle. *Child Abuse and Neglect, 8*, 203–217.

Nickman, S. (1985). Losses in adoption: The need for dialogue. *The Psychoanalytic Study of the Child, 40*, 365–398.

Novick, J., & Novick, C.K. (1991a). Scientific proceedings – Panel reports: Sadism and masochism in character disorder and resistance. *Journal of the American Psychoanalytic Association, 39*, 215–226.

Novick, J., & Novick, C.K. (1991b). Some comments on masochism and the delusion of omnipotence from a developmental perspective. *Journal of the American Psychoanalytic Association, 39*, 307–331.

Ornstein, A. (1991). Scientific proceedings – Panel reports: Sadism and masochism in character disorder and resistance. *Journal of the American Psychoanalytic Association, 39,* 215–226.

Pruett, C.D. (1984). A chronology of defensive adaptations to severe psychological trauma. *The Psychoanalytic Study of the Child, 39,* 591–612.

Pine, F. (1990). *Drive, ego, object & self: A synthesis for clinical work.* New York: Basic Books.

Raphael, B. (1983). *The anatomy of bereavement.* New York: Basic Books.

Rothstein, A. (1991). Sadomasochism in the neurosis conceived of as a pathological compromise formation. *Journal of the American Psychoanalytic Association, 39,* 363–375.

Rutter, M., & Quinton, D. (1984). Parental psychiatric disorder: Effects on children. *Psychological Medicine, 14,* 853–880.

Rutter, M. (1971). Parent–child separation: Psychological effects on the children. *Journal of Child Psychology and Psychiatry, 12,* 233–260.

Samaroff, A.J., Barocas, R., & Seifer, R. (1984). The early development of children born to mentally ill women. In N. Watt, E.J. Anthony, L. Wynne, & J. Rolf (Eds.), *Children at risk for schizophrenia* (pp. 482–514). New York: Cambridge University Press.

Seifer, R., & Samaroff, A. (1981). Adaptive behavior in young children of emotionally disturbed women. *Journal of Applied Developmental Psychology, I,* 251–276.

Smith, H.F. (1990). Cues: The perceptual edge of the transference. *International Journal of the Psychoanalytic Association, 71,* 219–228.

Stern, D. (1985). *The interpersonal world of the infant.* New York: Basic Books.

Weintraub, S. (1987). Risk factors in schizophrenia: The Stony Brook high-risk project. *Schizophrenia Bulletin, 13,* 439–449.

# Dyadic Circularity in the Mother–Infant Relationship

## ELIZABETH TUTERS

Infants are preprogrammed with a high capacity for perceptual discernment in interaction with their environment (Stern, 1985). The mother can also learn about her infant before birth by tracking the biological rhythms of the baby's activity and rest in the womb. Ideally, she does this naturally as a part of her necessary and increasing preoccupation with her infant (Winnicott, 1965). This dynamic primary relationship constitutes the first biopsychosocial ecology of the infant. In a way, the passage of the baby through the birth canal is a metaphor for the emergence of that relationship into the world, where it is influenced by and influences all future relationships.

As early as 1940, Donald Winnicott said: 'there is no such thing as an infant; meaning of course, that whenever one finds an infant, one finds maternal care, and without maternal care there would be no infant,' (cited in Winnicott, 1965, p. 39). In our present society, maternal care is no longer the exclusive relationship of mother–infant, but must be viewed as embracing both the parents and other caregivers who play a significant role in the child's life. However, the primary importance of relationships to the infant remains the same. In the case discussed below, caregivers include both community supports and the wider systems. The impact of these larger systems on the infant–mother dyad is also examined.

In infancy, the role of emotions is probably more significant than at any other age, as emotional signals serve as the language for the baby and are essential mediators in the infant–caregiver relationship (Emde, 1987). Emotions initiate and sustain social exchanges and seem vital for motivating engagement in the expanding world of infants interacting with caregivers, and caregivers interacting with infants.

Caregivers need to be cognizant of the interdependence of relationships that develop around any infant. These relationships are always affecting one another, and at the same time have an impact on the infant. A system that is sensitive to the influence of relationships upon relationships will ensure the emotional well-being of infants by valuing and supporting the complex matrix that exists. This is the very essence of quality caring, whether parental or non-parental (Emde, 1987).

**Infant Capacities**

Recent infant research has made the world aware of what experiences are like for infants and how competent infants are from birth (Stern, 1985). As Fraiberg, Adelson, and Shapiro (1980) have suggested, infants have strong self-righting tendencies and strong development functions – biologically based pathways that thrust towards sensory, motor, and social development. Paradoxically, babies are active, yet vulnerable participants in their own development; their very capacities increase their vulnerability to environmental failure. In fact, without environmental sensitivity to what a baby needs for optimal emotional well-being, the baby's innate capacities will cause him or her to adapt to an inappropriate and inadequate environment with long-standing deleterious effects. These effects are detrimental, not only to the baby, but to the baby in all relationships in the family and community.

Using these innate capacities, a baby processes ongoing experiences of the world, and gradually forms a sense of core self. For healthy development to occur, Stern (1985) suggested that an infant requires experiences of self-agency, self-coherency, self-history, and self-affectivity. These four basic experiences occur only within relationships; thus, the development of self is dependent on interactions with others. Self experiences are also interdependent, interrelated, and mutually reinforcing (Stern, 1985).

In an extension of his theory, Stern stated that infants have demonstrated the ability to take such subjective experiences of individual, specific events and interactions, and integrate them into an average representation, which he calls 'RIGS' (that is, representations of interactions that have been generalized). It has been suggested that this is an ongoing process beginning in the first year of life, which is used by the infant to organize experience and develop a sense of self. Since infants are entirely dependent on the care of others, caregiver responsiveness intimately affects all self-experience.

## Affect Attunement and Empathy

Caregivers and infants mutually create the chains and sequences of reciprocal behaviours that make up social dialogue during the child's early months. This phenomenon is called 'affect attunement.' A sense of subjective self is developed from intersubjective relatedness – that is, the relationship between self and other, through interaffectivity or shared feeling states (Stern, 1985).

Affect attunement, then, is expressed through interactions that convey a shared feeling state without simply imitating the exact behavioural expression of the inner state. There are three general features of behaviour that can be matched, and thereby form the basis of an attunement – namely, intensity, timing, and shape. Reflecting back an infant's feeling state is important to the infant's growing knowledge of his or her own feeling state and sense of self. Attunements occur largely outside awareness, and almost automatically. Affect attunement, which takes place spontaneously, is complemented by empathy, which requires a more deliberate thoughtfulness (Stern, 1985).

According to infant researcher Virginia Demos (1984), empathy has been defined as the act of putting oneself in the other's place, or entering into the other's state of mind. The development of empathy in adult caregivers requires that they develop capacities to: (1) resonate to the feeling states of the infant; (2) abstract knowledge from the experience of this emotional resonance; and (3) integrate the abstracted empathic knowledge into an empathic response (Stern, 1985, p. 145). The sequencing of these processes enables the caregiver to identify momentarily with the feeling state of the infant and to respond sensitively and appropriately to the infant's needs (in this case, the infant–mother pair needs).

The attunement of the caregiver to her own 'inner states' enables her to separate her own needs from those of the infant, and thus become more responsive to the infant–mother pair, while also recognizing and accepting her own feelings (Schwaber, 1984).

*Case History*

Sara, a rather fragile twenty-one-year-old woman, was three months pregnant when she was admitted to a home for single mothers, where she disclosed that she had been both physically and sexually abused by her father, as well as physically abused and rejected by her mother. She revealed she had attempted suicide five months previously, by running in front of a car. Sara was referred to a psychiatrist for supportive therapy, but refused to go. The staff felt concern for her ability to parent her baby.

Sara was the middle child in a sibline of three. She stated that she had never felt loved by her mother and had no memories of receiving affection. Although her father physically mistreated her, he also treated Sara with a 'special' affection throughout her childhood. Sara's family lived in a rural area and was known to the child welfare services. She was admitted to a psychiatric hospital when she was eight years old, with symptoms of anxiety and depression. Family therapy was attempted, but was discontinued as neither parent would commit to treatment. When Sara was sixteen years old, her parents separated. Sara's father was then hospitalized for approximately one month, with symptoms of severe depression. Sara had conscious memories of her father's sexual abuse following this hospitalization. Sara left home when her father began a relationship with another woman.

Sara had not seen her mother for several years. She claimed that her older sister was a prostitute whose two children had been apprehended by the child welfare services, and that her younger brother was a substance abuser. Sara herself did not have these problems.

When Sara left home, she lived with a violent young man. She gave birth to a male child, whom she placed for adoption. Sara's father was instrumental in having this baby relinquished to the child welfare services against her will. Sara attempted suicide after the baby was placed, and her boyfriend left her when she again became pregnant. She felt giving away the baby as giving away a part of herself, which she experienced as a trauma. She therefore replaced the lost baby with another.

Baby Martha was born one year later. Sara was living alone, and had had a difficult labour and delivery. Following the birth, Sara experienced extreme anxiety around her ability to parent. She worried that the authorities would take this baby away. With staff support, she sought help from the children's mental health agency to assist her with her parenting skills. She feared she might physically and sexually abuse her infant daughter. From the time Martha was one month old, both baby and mother were seen once a week by an infant mental health therapist to help Sara with her parenting skills. From birth, Martha suffered from problems digesting her formula. Sara could not breast-feed as she felt overstimulated and at risk of sexually abusing her daughter. Martha's digestion problem required hospitalization on two occasions. Martha's weight gain was slow and the hospital suspected non-organic failure-to-thrive. During her last hospitalization, Martha was found to have a medical problem, which required no intervention, only constant medical monitoring. Anxiety was expressed by all those working with this infant–mother pair because of the instability of the baby's weight and the unstable environmental situation.

During this early period, Sara moved homes several times. She went from home to hostel, to a housing project. Sara required a network of supports, owing to the nature of her difficulties and the high-risk situation for her and her infant daughter. A child welfare worker was assigned to her, and a public health nurse monitored the mother–infant relationship on a weekly basis. Sara also attended a parenting group and had ongoing contact with the hospital, where she was seen weekly for medical monitoring. The network required careful orchestration by the infant mental health therapist.

*The Treatment Process*

Developing and maintaining a parent–professional working alliance was crucial to the treatment process. Zeanah and McDonough (1989) have highlighted five interrelated clinical principles essential to developing these working alliances:

1 Sensitivity to the family's unique situation
2 Responsivity to the family's needs
3 Positive connotation to infant and parent behaviour
4 A non-judgmental attitude
5 A willingness to monitor intense feelings aroused by the family

Intervention with the mother–infant pair required that these five principles be kept in mind. The primary model of intervention used in this instance, conceptualized by N. Stern-Bruschweiler and D. Stern (1989), consisted of interactional coaching – that is, observing the interactive behaviour between infant and mother, and attempting to focus on the positive interactions observed in those behaviours. In addition, a psychoanalytic approach was used, where the therapist focused, when possible, on the mother's representational world in an attempt to connect her present situation and difficulties in relationship with her infant to her own past relational system.

The following is an example of interactional coaching: As Sara fed Martha, she told me about all the negative things her baby was doing. I noticed as she talked to me that Martha was looking up at her. I pointed out to Sara how intensely Martha was watching her; Sara seemed surprised. She looked down at Martha, who smiled up at her. Sara returned her smile and said to me, 'Look, she likes me!' At that point I validated her observation.

The following is an example of the psychoanalytic approach: Sara insisted her infant rejected her and was not interested in playing with her. This was connected with her own past experience of feeling rejected by her mother, who only hit her and never played with her as a child. Sara agreed no one had ever played with her. She herself did not know how to play; in fact, she continually waited to be hit by her infant with a toy.

The concept of intergenerational transmission of the abused–abusing pattern has been well substantiated in the literature (Main & Goldwyn, 1984). In this instance, the mother had been abused by both parents throughout her childhood. The infant research literature has suggested that the subjective experience of an infant (the infant's representational world) develops over time from interactions with caregivers (Stern, 1985). In this instance, Martha's representational world would be developed exclusively from her ongoing experience with her mother.

Sara sought help so that she would not physically or sexually abuse her baby. She revealed, through her observable behaviour with her infant, her inability to be attuned and to be sensitive to her infant. She was unable to read her infant's signals. As a child, Sara herself had not been attuned to herself; she had not been spoken to, played with, or nurtured by her own parents. The task of the therapy was to help Sara relate to her infant in a sensitive and enjoyable manner, so that her infant would thrive developmentally. The forty-five-minute sessions took place in a room with toys, with therapist, mother, and baby on the floor together. The therapist focused on the baby's relatedness to the mother and helped the mother understand the baby's communication to her mother and the mother's communication to the baby. Martha was early to develop and seemed precocious, which thrilled Sara, as it made her feel that she was being a good mother and her daughter would grow up soon to nurture her.

When things went well, Sara was delighted with Martha's development. However, if the baby became ill, Sara was upset and angry, and became fragmented. She exhibited incoherence and disorganization and was unable to comfort her upset baby. During these times, Sara behaved in a paranoid fashion, which was a concern and created ambivalence among members of the caring network. The caregivers struggled with the idea of removing the baby from the home, to have her in a place of safety. However, there was never sufficient evidence to apprehend the baby and, it was felt that, with ongoing support, Sara could reorganize herself and be more available for her infant. A working alliance had been established with the social worker from the child welfare agency, who then joined many of the therapy sessions at the mother's request.

The therapist had to struggle with her own anxiety in terms of the baby's safety, and used empathic listening to enable herself to be in touch with the mother's sensitivities and vulnerabilities. Sara was sensitive to the concerns of the support workers in her system, who she felt were looking for her to fail in her role as a mother. The therapist was aware of Sara's desire not to repeat her painful past and her wish to be a good mother for Martha, to give her what she had never been given herself. Sara had never had the experience of having her affective states affirmed by her own parents. Therefore, she had difficulty attuning to the affective states of her infant. Because of this lack of attunement in her own life, Sara lived in a state of self-fragmentation, which, under conditions of stress, affected her ability to think.

The therapist's ongoing attention to both the mother and infant, particularly the mother–infant dyad, provided a caring function for the mother. Sara experienced the therapist's empathic responsiveness as a functional component of her own self-organization. The mother began to internalize the therapist's empathic observational stance. Sara's understanding, accepting, and comforting attitude towards her infant's affective states paralleled her therapist's attitude with her – a process of identification with a new caring person.

## Summary

Of the many difficulties working with high-risk cases of infant–mother relationships, the greatest challenge was dealing with the anxiety created in all members of the caregiver system. The aim of the intervention was to help the mother develop the capacity to meet her infant's needs, and in so doing, this mother, who had been so deprived in her own life, had her own needs met as her infant developed into a confident, exploring toddler.

The objective of the intervention was to effect changes in the mother's representational world and relational system in order to interrupt the intergenerational transmission of abuse and neglect. The infant has continued to grow and to develop a strong affective sense of self – as the mother has understood her own issues through the tie with the therapist, and the tie with the social worker in the child welfare agency and the others in the supportive network. It was the clinician's task to maintain a therapeutic alliance with all members of the support system in order to help this high-risk mother achieve optimal mental health for her child.

REFERENCES

Demos, V. (1984). Empathy and affect: Reflections of infant experience. In J. Lichtenberg, M. Bornstein, & D. Silver (Eds.), *Empathy II* (pp. 9–34). Hillsdale, NJ: Analytic Press.

Emde, R. (1987). Infant mental health: Clinical dilemmas, the expansion of meaning and opportunities. In J. Osofsky (Ed.), *Handbook of infant development* (2d ed.) (pp. 1297–1321). New York: Wiley & Sons.

Fraiberg, S., Adelson, E., & Shapiro, V. (1980). Ghosts in the nursery, In S. Fraiberg (Ed.), *Clinical studies in infant mental health* (pp. 169–194). New York: Basic Books.

Main, M., & Goldwyn, R. (1984). Predicting rejection of her infant from mother representation of her own experience: Implications for the abused-abusing intergenerational cycle. *Child Abuse and Neglect, 8,* 203–217.

Schwaber, E. (1984). Empathy: A mode of analytic listening. In J. Lichtenberg, M. Bornstein, & D. Silver (Eds.), *Empathy II* (pp. 143–172). Hillsdale, NJ: Analytic Press.

Stern, D. (1985). *The interpersonal world of the infant.* New York: Basic Books

Stern-Bruschweiler, N., & Stern, D. (1989). A model for conceptualizing the role of the mother's representational world in various mother–infant therapies. *Infant Mental Health Journal, 10* (3), 142–156.

Tuters, E. (1988). The relevance of infant observation to clinical training and practice: An interpretation. *Infant Mental Health Journal, 9* (1), 93–104.

Winnicott, D.W. (1965). The theory of the parent–infant relationship. In D.W. Winnicott (Ed.), *The maturational process and the facilitating environment* (pp. 37–55). London: Hogarth Press.

Zeanah, C., & McDonough, S. (1989). Clinical approaches to families in early intervention. *Seminars in Perinatology, 13,* 513–522.